Biomedicine as Culture

Routledge Studies in Science, Technology and Society

Biomedicine as Culture

Instrumental Practices, Technoscientific
Knowledge, and New Modes of Life

Edited by
Regula Valérie Burri
and Joseph Dumit

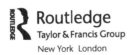
Routledge
Taylor & Francis Group
New York London

Routledge
Taylor & Francis Group
605 Third Avenue,
New York, NY 10017

Routledge
Taylor & Francis Group
2 Park Square
Milton Park, Abingdon
Oxon OX14 4RN

© 2007 by Taylor & Francis
Routledge is an imprint of Taylor & Francis Group, an Informa business

---

Library of Congress Cataloging-in-Publication Data

Biomedicine as culture : instrumental practices, technoscientific knowledge, and new
  modes of life / edited by Regula Valérie Burri and Joseph Dumit.
      p. ; cm. -- (Routledge studies in science, technology, and society ; 6)
  Includes bibliographical references and index.
  ISBN 978-0-415-95798-4 (hardback : alk. paper)
  1. Medicine--Philosophy. 2. Social medicine. 3. Medical anthropology. I. Burri,
Regula Valérie. II. Dumit, Joseph. III. Series.
  [DNLM: 1. Sociology, Medical. 2. Anthropology, Cultural. 3. Culture. 4.
Philosophy, Medical. WA 31 B615 2007]

  R723.B535 2007
  610.28--dc22
                                                                    2006101206

ISBN 13: 978-0-415-88317-7 (pbk)
ISBN 13: 978-0-415-95798-4 (hbk)

Contents

Foreword

In recent years, scientific and technological innovations, changes in societal structures and attitudes, as well as budgetary restrictions have been forcing a reorientation in medicine. Societal demands for cutting-edge health care and provision contrast with ethical dilemmas and scarce finances in a health system that is increasingly cost-intensive. The economic dominance of the health care discourse together with insufficient communications between the different stakeholders in the medical field and an increasing social resistance to an alienated academic medicine foster the need to rethink medicine and its future, and reconsider its values and goals. As part of its long-term engagement in this process, the Swiss Academy of Medical Sciences entered into dialogue with researchers from the social sciences and humanities. Together with its sister academy—the Swiss Academy of Humanities and Social Sciences—it initiated a first joint symposium to discuss medicine from a social science point of view. Entitled "Medicine as Culture: Cultural Studies of Medicine," the resulting international conference, organized by Regula Valérie Burri, Margrit Leuthold, Viviane von Kaenel, and Markus Zürcher, took place in Zurich in November 2004. It included speakers from Europe, the United States, and Canada who represented a variety of disciplines. The papers of this conference are included in this collection, which discusses (bio)medicine's current practices and offers a critical assessment of their social and cultural implications.

Dr. Margrit Leuthold
Swiss Academy of Medical Sciences (SAMS)

Dr. Markus Zürcher
Swiss Academy of Humanities and Social Sciences (SAHS)

Introduction

Regula Valérie Burri and Joseph Dumit

While the study of "medicine and culture" has a long tradition within social studies and the humanities (e.g., medical anthropology, medical sociology, and history and philosophy of medicine), this volume examines "(bio-)medicine as culture" from a contemporary, science studies-based perspective. It reflects the growing impact of technology in medical research and routine practices and their increasing intertwinedness with other life sciences like genomics or neurosciences.[1] This perspective engages new questions regarding the relation between biomedicine and its cultural context, which implies new dynamics between local and global worlds of knowledge, technology, and practice (Good 1995, 2001). The genetic assumptions of biomedicine reconfigure the boundaries not only between nature and culture in the life sciences but also in society in general when reencoding the categories of health and illness, of normality and pathology. At the same time, predictive diagnostic methods become more and more important. Speaking of "genetic risks" and "genetic responsibility" raises fundamental questions about cultural backgrounds of biomedical practices and its consequences for society and people's identities, bringing up issues of "emergent forms of life" (Fischer 2003; Rose, this volume).

Our collection of essays takes up some of these questions. Following the practice turn in social theory (Schatzki et al. 2001; Bourdieu 1972/2002, 1980/1992), the volume examines practices of biomedical knowledge production and looks at the ways they reencode material cultures, epistemic orders, and social configurations—both within and outside the laboratories and clinics. This perspective implies that biomedical practices are situated in the context of the larger developments in science, medicine, and society; many science and technology studies (STS) scholars have shown how biomedical knowledge production is embedded in and shaped by cultural contexts (e.g., Fujimura 1996; Clarke 1998). Three major and intertwined processes can be distinguished when looking at the transformations in recent health care production and provision: scientification of biomedicine, socialization of biomedicine, and biomedicalization of society.

SCIENTIFICATION OF BIOMEDICINE

Medicine has been undergoing major transformations during the last two decades. New scientific and technological advancements have been influential in changing the ways medical knowledge is produced and applied in laboratories and hospitals today. Medicine has increasingly been converging with other life sciences such as molecular biology and neurosciences while at the same time drawing on physical, chemical, and computer sciences. The molecularization of biology and medicine can be traced back to the beginnings of the last century (de Chadarevian & Kamminga 1998), but recent medical technologies and methods like biotechnology, genomics, bioinformatics, and imaging technology have been providing new material tools and procedures for diagnosis and treatment. This has not only altered the epistemic foundations of knowledge production in medicine but also dramatically changed the ways in which this knowledge is produced, distributed, and applied. Since the 1950s, the consequences of the transformation of medicine into biomedicine have involved major reconfigurations in health care—ranging from the ways illnesses are defined or bodies are seen to therapeutic interventions to hospital architecture. Peter Keating and Alberto Cambrosio (2003) have reconstructed how such configurations of instruments, social actors, and medical programs—so-called biomedical platforms—have been transformed in this period, thus entailing a new alignment between the normal and the pathological. Adele Clarke and co-authors (Clarke, Fishman et al. 2000; Clarke, Shim et al. 2003) used the term *biomedicalization* to point to the integration of technoscientific innovations in medicine since the mid-1980s and underlined that it goes along with new social forms and organizational infrastructures, with new practices of contemporary biomedicine, and with a shift from the control over biomedical phenomena to transformations of them. Biomedicalization also shifts the focus of biomedical practices from healing to health itself when enhancement of bodily functions and conditions becomes the target of medical research and interventions.

In *Differences in Medicine* (1998), editors Marc Berg and Annemarie Mol showed that medicine is not to be considered as something homogeneous but consists of a multiplicity of local negotiations and contingent practices. Diagnostic knowledge, medical treatments, and the patients' bodies, the authors analyzed, thus have to be seen as discontinuous entities shaped in specific contexts. The heterogeneity of medical knowledge and everyday practices has also been an object of concern within the medical community. Epidemiologists have criticized the lack of scientific substantiations in daily medical practice and claimed an evidence-based medicine which grounds medical decision making on scientific principles and clinical research and which leads to an increasing standardization of medical practice (cf. Timmermans & Berg 2003). This turn toward randomized clinical trials and the elaboration of clinical practice guidelines based on an assessment of scientific literature is one of the most prominent recent manifestations of the rationalization of medicine (Timmermans 2005). Decision-support techniques like protocols or expert systems have transformed medical work (Berg 1997), and clinical trials research "vested in new bioinformatics and biostatistics continuously redefines both the content of health interventions (e.g., by defining 'unnecessary' treatments) and the scientific criteria of medical knowledge production by standardizing drug evaluation" (Timmermans 2005: 326).

The scientification of biomedicine thus implies both the increasing intertwinedness of medicine with science and its technological innovations and the growing implementation of a science-based process of rationalization in medicine. Together, these processes reconfigure the epistemic tools, the material procedures, and the social relations and infrastructures in biomedicine and exert a major impact on society in general.

SOCIALIZATION OF BIOMEDICINE

While the scientification of biomedicine is focused on the prevalence of science in medicine, the "socialization of biomedicine" refers to the processes by which society gets involved in medical knowledge production and diffusion. In recent years, the public calling into question of scientific authority has challenged the relations between scientific experts and laypeople and contributed to the emergence of new modes of knowledge production (Gibbons et al. 1994; Nowotny et al. 2001). In medicine, these changes, along with patients' better access to relevant medical information through the Internet (which enabled the organization of patient groups), have fostered the active participation of laypeople in research (see also Taussig and Oudshoorn & Somers, this volume). In his study on the U.S. AIDS activists' movement in the 1980s, Steven Epstein (1996) has traced the ways activists participated in the debates on the causes of AIDS and the search for possible treatments of it. He showed how in the course of the development of AIDS research, lay expertise gained credibility within the scientific community and played a significant role in medical research when influencing the methods used in clinical drug trials. Vololona Rabeharisoa and Michel Callon (2002, 2004) studied the involvement of patients' associations in research on muscular dystrophy in France. Rabeharisoa (2003) distinguished three different types of patient organizations' engagement in research which each imply specific power relations between patients and professionals. In contrast to the classic "auxiliary model" in which the patient organizations mostly rely on specialists to take decisions on the research orientations, and the "emancipatory model" in which the organizations claim patients' strong participation in decisions concerning them—and even sometimes try to free themselves from any expertise that does not derive from their own experiences—the "partnership model" found in the organization involved in muscular dystrophy research is based on a different concept of the relation between experts and laypeople. In this model, patient organizations are masters of the research policy on the respective illnesses and patients are considered partners in their own right.

Such collaborations between scientists and patient groups are emerging forms of science–society interactions. They shape new ways of scientific knowledge production by integrating different actors, methods, and experiences, and they also contribute to a distinctive way of thinking about the inclusion of women, racial and ethnic minorities, children, and the elderly as research subjects (Epstein, forthcoming). In biomedicine, "researchers in the wild" (Callon & Rabeharisoa 2003) meet with laboratory workers and practitioners, and they all are involved in the negotiation of what is considered as legitimate knowledge. The collective forms of research change social relations and institutional arrangements, and, as Callon and Rabeharisoa show, also coproduce patients' identities.

BIOMEDICALIZATION OF SOCIETY

The processes described so far relate to the role of science and society in medicine; "biomedicalization of society" refers to the opposite process of the transformations of society induced by biomedicine. Since the middle of the last century, a growing number of aspects of life have become defined as medical problems. This expansion of medical jurisdiction has been described as "medicalization" (Zola 1972; Conrad 1992; Clarke, Shim et al. 2003; see also Beck, this volume). Through medicalization, a medical perspective increasingly applies to realms which have not been considered as medical before. Recently, the scientification of medicine has dramatically enforced and accelerated this process and provoked radical changes by reconfiguring social orders and identities. Life itself has become subject to new modes of intervention and governance which created a new form of genetic and biological citizenship (Rapp & Ginsburg 2001; Rose & Novas 2004; Rose 2001, 2006, and this volume). Increasingly, human relations and decisions rely on a consciousness focused on the maintenance and improvement of health and human conditions. Illnesses are "invented," and new "pharmaceutical" ways of thinking emerge (Young 1995; Lakoff 2005). Health has become a moral responsibility when the management of illnesses and health risks is defined as a personal duty to be fulfilled (cf. Rose and Lemke, this volume).

Statistical models of risk and probabilities as well as new genetic knowledge and emerging technologies have to be incorporated and handled within daily life, and they become part of everyday conversations (cf. Duden & Samerski and Taussig, this volume). Charis Cussins (1998) has shown that the objectification, naturalization, and bureaucratization implied in such confrontations with technoscience do not necessarily entail being helpless or being a victim. Based on her field research in an infertility clinic she demonstrates that women patients do not generally lose their agency when making use of new medical technologies but rather pursue agency and become a self by their active participation in the treatments. Rayna Rapp (1999) pointed to the differences in such "living by numbers" when examining the social impact of amniocentesis in the United States. She showed how women in daily life brought together the new genetics with their understandings of motherhood and kinship differently, depending on their social background.

The entangled nature of biomedical knowledge and technology in everyday life encompasses the transformation of how the body is constructed, seen, and talked about. Aesthetic surgery and pharmaceutical drugs to enhance cognitive functions both come along with growing cultural impositions to individually shape and improve personal bodies. Studying the changing discourse on the immune system in the United States, Emily Martin (1994) reveals how emergent views of the body as a flexible system imply concepts of a new social Darwinism by which some people are seen as more flexible and adaptable than others, according to the quality of their immune system, and hence are considered as occupying a different rank in society. Such ascriptions and the formation of new social groups and institutions on the basis of technoscientific knowledge comprise the most prominent social reconfigurations induced by the recent developments in biomedical research. New reproduction technologies, for example, have created new forms of family and kinship relations (e.g., Strathern 1992; Franklin 1997; Edwards et al. 1993/1999; Franklin & McKinnon 2001; Thompson 2005). Genetic testing, as another example, restructures social orders and individual persons when identifying individuals and groups with potential risks for certain illnesses (cf. Rose; Lemke; Duden & Samerski, this volume). Paul Rabinow (1992, 1996) formulated the concept of biosociality to suggest the emergence of such new social communities around particular biological conditions, and to describe the shift from a sociobiological culture which is modeled on nature to the culturalization and engineering of nature itself. These reconfigurations are intertwined with a global industrial complex. Global biocapital and transnational economic markets and interests—as well as different regulatory regimes (Jasanoff 2005)—are involved in the shaping of research orientations and the ways health care is produced and provided (e.g., Krimsky 2003; Franklin & Lock 2003; Franklin 2005; Greenslit 2005; Martin 2006; Petryna et al. 2006; Sunder Rajan 2006; Waldby & Mitchell 2006; Rose, this volume). From these processes of biomedicalization that converge with other sociotechnical developments, specific "bioscapes" (Dumit & Burri, this volume) emerge that will challenge society in the future.

Our volume follows up on some of these features. It offers interdisciplinary perspectives on contemporary biomedicine as a cultural practice. The collection of essays brings together leading scholars from cultural anthropology, sociology, history, and science studies to conduct a critical dialogue on the culture(s) of biomedical practice, discussing its epistemic, material, and social implications. The essays look at the ways new biomedical knowledge is constructed within hospitals and academic settings and at how this knowledge changes perceptions, material arrangements, and social relations not only within clinics and scientific communities but also especially once it is diffused into a broader cultural context.[2]

The volume consists of three sections: part I discusses theoretical and disciplinary approaches to the study of biomedicine as culture, part II focuses on knowledge practices within research communities and clinical settings, and part III explores the transformations in society induced by this new generated knowledge.

Following this introduction, the first section, "Social and cultural studies of biomedicine," focuses on theoretical concepts and methodological approaches that sociology, cultural anthropology, history, and science studies can offer to the study of contemporary biomedicine. Stefan Beck's chapter, "Medicalizing culture(s) or culturalizing medicine(s)," opens the volume with a discussion of the key concept of "medicalization" as an often used but—as Beck argues—not entirely adequate category for the anthropological analysis of contemporary biomedicine. Taking a case study on the Bone Marrow Donor Registry in Cyprus as a starting point for reflection, Beck shows how the implementation of biomedical knowledge is sensitive to the local culture and implies the adoption of medical options and technologies on the part of the involved subjects. The essay suggests understanding the diversity, heterogeneity, and complexity of biomedical epistemic practices and effects in their dynamic cultural contexts; looking at the interdependencies of the "social" and the "biological"; and analyzing the ways scientific practices, social norms, material structures, administrative routines, value systems, and legal regimes are locally assembled and negotiated. Jakob Tanner's essay, "Metaphors of medicine and the culture of healing: Historical perspectives," offers a critical reading of historical understandings of biomedicine as culture. The essay elaborates on the use of metaphors in medicine and outlines four crucial questions of current historical interest in the field: (1) the forms of knowledge and (bio-)power as they become manifest in biopolitical mechanisms; (2) the semiotics adopted by medical experts to integrate heterogeneous clinical indications and signs into a coherent framework of interpretation; (3) the cross-cultural comparison of "medical systems" and therapeutic practices; and (4) the transformations of diagnostic classifications and subjective experience through new clinical procedures and therapeutic trajectories. Gesa Lindemann takes a completely different perspective. Her essay, "Medicine as practice and culture: The analysis of border regimes and the necessity of a hermeneutics of physical bodies," suggests conceptualizing biomedicine as a "new border regime" that defines—because of its contingent classifications of life and death—the demarcations of what is culturally considered a social actor. Drawing on gestalt theory and field research in intensive care units in Germany, Lindemann develops a methodology to analyze physicians' practices and patients' bodies in the interactional situation. Following the arguments in this first section, social or cultural studies of biomedicine provide an important input to social theory in general.

The second section, "Epistemic practices and material culture(s)," examines how biomedical knowledge is socially and historically produced and renegotiated within biomedical research and clinical practice. This involves actors, ideas, technologies, and bodies that are constantly constituted and reconfigured during the knowledge generation processes. In the first chapter, "The future is now: Locating biomarkers for dementia," Margaret Lock focuses on scientists' search for genetic "biomarkers" to predict Alzheimer's disease. Her essay situates the "discovery" of mild cognitive impairment in the early 1990s within the history of genetics, which is described as a shift from a conception of heredity to genetic determinism to a view where biological pathways are no longer understood as being unidirectional. In search of the causes for prodromal dementia, researchers concentrate on the detection of "biomarkers" which are thought of as the core, or essence, of Alzheimer's disease and as being—besides age—a major risk factor. This view, the essay argues, is a regression on individualized thinking about dementia causality and neglects other causes such as environmental effects. The essay reviews the practices to detect biomarkers aimed at establishing clear boundaries for prodromal dementia by critically exploring some of the effects of informing individuals about genetic test results. Annemarie Mol and John Law's essay, "Embodied action, enacted bodies: The example of hypoglycaemia," looks at material and epistemic practices by theorizing how the patient's body is constituted and enacted when handling and living with diabetes. Including text materials, interviews and ethnographic field observations made in medical clinics in the Netherlands, and arguing from a philosophical and science studies point of view, the essay asks how the body is known and enacted in current medical practices. Not understanding hypoglycaemia as hidden in the body or beneath the skin but as enacted by the acting body, the essay points to the coeval processes by which the body is being performed or done. It argues that by practices of measuring, watching, intervening, feeling, counteracting, and avoiding, the hypoglycemic body is both acting and being enacted at the same time. Regula Valérie Burri's contribution analyzes the "Socio-technical anatomy" that underlies the process of the production of visual medical knowledge in biomedical practice. The essay explores the interplay of technological apparatuses, institutional and spatial arrangements, physicians, bodies, diagnostic interpretations, and implicit knowledge in the process of image production. Drawing on multisited ethnographic field research in several Magnetic Resonance Imaging Units in Switzerland, Germany, and the United States, the essay shows how the material cultures and epistemic practices in the process of image fabrication all contribute to a (re-)constitution of "instrumental bodies"—bodies that are prepared and made instrumental in order to enable the production of a medical image. Cornelius Schubert's essay, "Risk and safety in the operating theater: An ethnographic study of sociotechnical practices," undertakes a study of anesthetic practices, focusing on safety and cooperation in surgical operating rooms. Based on video observations and fieldwork in several German and Australian hospitals and drawing from technology and workplace studies, the essay analyzes the practices of anesthetists displayed in local situations. It identifies the specific elements constituting local patterns of cooperation by examining the daily activities and work routines directed to patients' safety, thus offering a model to analyze these safety-relevant practices.

The third section, "Biomedical knowledge in context," considers the reconfigurations induced by recent biomedical research in society in general. It looks at how cultural perceptions, people's identities and agency, social relations and institutions, as well as technical equipments are transformed by new medical discourses and methods. Nikolas Rose's chapter, "Genomic susceptibility as an emergent form of life? Genetic testing, identity, and the remit of medicine," opens the section with a discussion on potential social consequences of the increasing ability of genetic testing to identify susceptibilities to disease prior to the appearance of symptoms. It explores how these developments are contributing to an "emergent form of life" which takes shape in the new sets of relations between biomedical research and private corporations that aim at extracting value from the very vital character of human life itself. This search for "biovalue," the essay argues, not only shapes diagnostic categories—when their expansion goes hand in hand with the development and selling of pharmaceuticals—but also leads to the rise of a new style of thought that extends the power of biomedicine to the management of life itself by imposing on susceptible individuals the obligation to actively handle the illnesses they might get in the future. Thomas Lemke's essay, "Susceptible individuals and risky rights: Dimensions of genetic responsibility," follows up on this topic. Drawing on legal cases from the United States, it points to the emergence of a discourse of "genetic responsibility" which is currently shaping judicial decisions. The essay shows how this discourse is concerned with reproductive decisions to prevent diseases and with the obligation both to communicate genetic information to family members "at risk" and to control one's own potential diseases by informed choices of lifestyle options. New genetic knowledge, the essay argues, thus engenders new modes of responsible agency and is made into a central point of reference to expand moral duties. Barbara Duden and Silja Samerski's contribution, "'Pop genes': An investigation of 'the gene' in popular parlance," examines the popular understanding and daily usage of new genetic knowledge and language. Based on fieldwork in a small German village and in genetic counseling sessions, it explores the adoption of the notions "gene" and "genetics" in everyday conversations and in talks between experts and laypeople. The essay points to the power of these words, which merge the most intimate aspects of a person—the soma—with statistical probabilities and risks. It argues that the symbolic meanings and fallouts of popular gene talk imply the potency of irreversibly transforming the individual subject.

The final two essays address how laypeople react to new biomedical knowledge, either rejecting it or acquiring and adopting it as a form of empowerment. The essays show how biomedical knowledge is used by patients, self-help groups, and people's organizations in order to build alliances and foster political action aimed at improving their health situation. Karen-Sue Taussig's essay, "Genetics and its publics: Crafting genetic literacy and identity in the early twenty-first century," looks at several education efforts to inform laypeople on genetic knowledge. By such education, the essay assumes, scientists hope to gain access to the material means—DNA, blood and tissue samples, family histories, and medical records—that are needed for the development of genomic medicine. By drawing on examples like a couple who started to build up a huge database on an inherited skin degeneration in the United States and now controls important research materials, or an Indigenous People's Council that declined to make available genetic resources, the essay points to the different uses of new biomedical knowledge and sketches some of the diverse social practices by which individuals are configured into biosocial citizens. Nelly Oudshoorn and André Somers's chapter, "Constructing the digital patient: Patient organizations and the development of health websites," finally asks in what way laypeople's agency is shaped by the specific construction and use of patient organizations' Internet websites. Based on a case study in the Netherlands, the essay demonstrates a variety of ways—from democratic to paternalistic—to design and manage such websites, and discusses the implications for patients' empowerment. By examining three different patient organizations, the essay shows how their health websites contribute to a redefinition of the patient from a passive actor toward one who is an active participant in his or her care.

In an epilogue, Joseph Dumit and Regula Valérie Burri offer a reading of the essays assembled in this volume in the context of emergent "bioscapes." They show how the convergence of biomedical innovations, information technologies, industrialized life sciences, and corporate clinical trials create terrains that are characterized by indetermination, standardization, postmedical demands, partial evidence, and logics of obligation.

NOTES

Acknowledgements. Our warmest thanks to Benjamin Holtzman, Routledge research editor, for being very helpful and making the publishing process go smoothly. We also thank Caroline Wiedmer for conversations about this project, the anonymous reviewers for their comments, and Cheryl Adam and Lynn Goeller

10   *Regula Valérie Burri and Joseph Dumit*

for copyediting the manuscript, and we are grateful to the Swiss Academies of Humanities and Social Sciences (SAHS) and of Medical Sciences (SAMS) for supporting this project.

1. In contrast to our volume, Deborah Lupton's (1994) *Medicine as Culture* takes approaches from medical sociology, sociology of health and illness, medical anthropology, and cultural studies to examine the sociocultural dimensions of medicine in Western society, and is thus—like many important works in medical anthropology (e.g., Good 1994; Kleinman 1997)—concerned with what we here call medicine *and* culture. Our volume draws from Margaret Lock and Deborah Gordon's (1988) *Biomedicine examined*, which was one of the first collections with a focus on the production and the cultural implications of biomedical knowledge.
2. Other collections of essays or monographs that discuss recent advances in biomedicine and apply a science studies perspective focus on the life sciences in general (e.g., Franklin & Lock 2003; Gaudillière & Rheinberger 2004; M'Charek 2005), on genetics exclusively (Fortun & Mendelsohn 1999; Goodman et al. 2003; Kerr 2004; Bunton & Petersen 2005), on medical technologies (Lock, Young et al. 2000; Lauritzen & Hyden 2006) and the risks of medical innovation (Schlich & Troehler 2006), on human organs (Hogle 1999; Lock 2002), or on selected diseases or procedures (e.g., pharmacogenomics: Hedgecoe 2004; immunophenotyping: Keating & Cambrosio 2003; Huntington's disease: Konrad 2005; cancer therapy: Löwy 1997; medical imaging: Dumit 2004; or reproductive technologies: Davis-Floyd & Dumit 1998; Rapp 1999; Becker 2000; Inhorn & van Balen 2002; Thompson 2005; Franklin & Roberts 2006). Several works in medical anthropology integrate a variety of approaches but do not primarily employ a science studies perspective (e.g., Sargent & Johnson 1996; Nichter & Lock 2002; Scheper-Hughes & Wacquant 2003). Other collections do apply such a perspective but because of their publication date were not able to integrate recent advances in biomedicine (Lock & Gordon 1988; Lachmund & Stollberg 1992; Berg & Mol 1998).

REFERENCES

Becker, Gay. 2000. *The elusive embryo: How women and men approach new reproductive technologies*. Berkeley: University of California Press.
Berg, Marc. 1997. *Rationalizing medical work: Decision-support techniques and medical practices*. Cambridge, MA: MIT Press.
Berg, Marc, and Annemarie Mol, eds. 1998. *Differences in medicine: Unraveling practices, techniques and bodies*. Durham, NC: Duke University Press.
Bourdieu, Pierre. 1972/2002. *Outline of a theory of practice*. Cambridge Studies in Social Anthropology, 16. Cambridge: Cambridge University Press.
———. 1980/1992. *The logic of practice*. Stanford, CA: Stanford University Press.
Bunton, Robin, and Alan Petersen, eds. 2005. *Genetic governance: Health, risk, and ethics in the biotech age*. London: Routledge.
Callon, Michel, and Vololona Rabeharisoa. 2003. Research "in the wild" and the shaping of new social identities. *Technology in Society* 25, no. 2: 193–204.
Clarke, Adele E. 1998. *Disciplining reproduction: Modernity, American life sciences, and the problems of sex*. Berkeley: University of California Press.

Clarke, Adele E., Jennifer R. Fishman, Jennifer Ruth Fosket, Laura Mamo, and Janet K. Shim. 2000. Technoscience and the new biomedicalization: Western roots, global rhizomes. *Sciences sociales et santé* 18, no. 2: 11–42.

Clarke, Adele E., Janet K. Shim, Laura Mamo, Jennifer Ruth Fosket, and Jennifer R. Fishman. 2003. Biomedicalization: Technoscientific transformations of health, illness, and U.S. biomedicine. *American Sociological Review* 68:161–94.

Conrad, Peter. 1992. Medicalization and social control. *Annual Review of Sociology* 18:209–32.

Cussins, Charis. 1998. Ontological choreography: Agency for women patients in an infertility clinic. In *Differences in medicine: Unraveling practices, techniques and bodies*, edited by Marc Berg and Annemarie Mol, 166–201. Durham, NC: Duke University Press.

Davis-Floyd, Robbie, and Joseph Dumit, eds. 1998. *Cyborg babies: From techno-sex to techno-tots.* London: Routledge.

de Chadarevian, Soraya, and Harmke Kamminga, eds. 1998. *Molecularizing biology and medicine: New alliances 1910s–1970s.* Amsterdam: Harwood Academic.

Dumit, Joseph. 2004. *Picturing personhood: Brain scans and biomedical identity.* Princeton, NJ: Princeton University Press.

Edwards, Jeanette, Sarah Franklin, Eric Hirsch, Frances Price, and Marilyn Strathern. 1993/1999. *Technologies of procreation: Kinship in the age of assisted conception.* London: Routledge.

Epstein, Steven. 1996. *Impure science: AIDS, activism, and the politics of knowledge.* Berkeley: University of California Press.

———. forthcoming. *Inclusion: The politics of difference in medical research.* Chicago: University of Chicago Press.

Fischer, Michael M. J. 2003. *Emergent forms of life and the anthropological voice.* Durham, NC: Duke University Press.

Fortun, Michael, and Everett Mendelsohn, eds. 1999. The practices of human genetics. *Sociology of the Sciences Yearbook,* vol. 21. Dordrecht: Kluwer Academic.

Franklin, Sarah. 1997. *Embodied progress: A cultural account of assisted conception.* London: Routledge.

———. 2005. Stem Cells R Us: Emergent life forms and the global biological. In *Global assemblages: Technology, politics, and ethics as anthropological problems*, edited by Aihwa Ong and Stephen Collier, 59–78. Oxford: Blackwell.

Franklin, Sarah, and Margaret M. Lock, eds. 2003. *Remaking life & death: Towards an anthropology of the biosciences.* Santa Fe, NM: SAR Press.

Franklin, Sarah, and Susan McKinnon, eds. 2001. *Relative values: Reconfiguring kinship studies.* Durham, NC: Duke University Press.

Franklin, Sarah, and Celia Roberts. 2006. *Born and made: An ethnography of pre-implantation genetic diagnosis.* Princeton, NJ: Princeton University Press.

Fujimura, Joan. 1996. *Crafting science: A socio-history of the quest for the genetics of cancer.* Cambridge, MA: Harvard University Press.

Gaudillière, Jean-Paul, and Hans-Jörg Rheinberger, eds. 2004. *From molecular genetics to genomics.* London: Routledge.

Gibbons, Michael, Helga Nowotny et al. 1994. *The new production of knowledge: The dynamics of science and research in contemporary societies.* London: Sage.

Good, Byron J. 1994. *Medicine, rationality and experience: An anthropological perspective.* Lewis Henry Morgan Lectures. Cambridge: Cambridge University Press.

Good, Mary-Jo DelVecchio. 1995. Cultural studies of biomedicine: An agenda for research. *Social Science and Medicine* 41, no. 4: 461–73.

———. 2001. The biotechnical embrace. *Culture, Medicine and Psychiatry* 25, no. 4: 395–410.

Goodman, Alan H., Deborah Heath, and Susan Lindee, eds. 2003. *Genetic nature/culture: Anthropology and science beyond the two-culture divide.* Berkeley: University of California Press.

Greenslit, Nathan. 2005. Depression and consumption: Psychopharmaceuticals, branding, and new identity practices. *Culture, Medicine and Psychiatry* 29, no. 4: 477–502.

Hedgecoe, Adam. 2004. *The politics of personalised medicine: Pharmacogenetics in the clinic.* Cambridge Studies in Society and the Life Sciences. Cambridge: Cambridge University Press.

Hogle, Linda. 1999. *Recovering the nation's body: Cultural memory, medicine, and the politics of redemption.* Piscataway, NJ: Rutgers University Press.

Inhorn, Marcia C., and Frank van Balen, eds. 2002. *Infertility around the globe: New thinking on childlessness, gender, and reproductive technologies.* Berkeley: University of California Press.

Jasanoff, Sheila. 2005. *Designs on nature: Science and democracy in Europe and the United States.* Princeton, NJ: Princeton University Press.

Keating, Peter, and Alberto Cambrosio. 2003. *Biomedical platforms: Realigning the normal and the pathological in late-twentieth-century medicine.* Cambridge, MA: MIT Press.

Kerr, Anne. 2004. *Genetics and society: A sociology of disease.* London: Routledge.

Kleinman, Arthur. 1997. *Writing at the margin: Discourse between anthropology and medicine.* Berkeley: University of California Press.

Konrad, Monica. 2005. *Narrating the new predictive genetics: Ethics, ethnography and science.* Cambridge Studies in Society and the Life Sciences. Cambridge: Cambridge University Press.

Krimsky, Sheldon. 2003. *Science in the private interest: Has the lure of profits corrupted biomedical research?* Lanham, MD: Rowman & Littlefield.

Lachmund, Jens, and Gunnar Stollberg, eds. 1992. *The social construction of illness: Illness and medical knowledge in past and present.* Stuttgart: Steiner.

Lakoff, Andrew. 2005. *Pharmaceutical reason: Knowledge and value in global psychiatry.* Cambridge Studies in Society and the Life Sciences. Cambridge: Cambridge University Press.

Lauritzen, Sonia Olin, and Lars-Christer Hyden, eds. 2006. *Medical technologies and the life worlds: The social construction of normality.* New York: Routledge.

Lock, Margaret. 2002. *Twice dead: Organ transplants and the reinvention of death.* Berkeley: University of California Press.

Lock, Margaret, and Deborah R. Gordon, eds. 1988. *Biomedicine examined.* Dordrecht: Kluwer Academic.

Lock, Margaret, Allan Young, and Alberto Cambrosio, eds. 2000. *Living and working with the new medical technologies: Intersections of inquiry.* Cambridge Studies in Medical Anthropology. Cambridge: Cambridge University Press.

Löwy, Ilana. 1997. *Between bench and bedside: Science, healing, and interleukin-2 in a cancer ward.* Cambridge, MA: Harvard University Press.

Lupton, Deborah. 1994. *Medicine as culture: Illness, disease and the body in Western society.* London: Sage.

Martin, Emily. 1994. *Flexible bodies: Tracking immunity in American culture—from the days of polio to the age of AIDS.* Boston: Beacon.

———. 2006. Pharmaceutical virtue. *Culture, Medicine and Psychiatry* 30, no. 2: 157–74.

M'Charek, Amade. 2005. *The Human Genome Diversity Project: An ethnography of scientific practice.* Cambridge Studies in Society and the Life Sciences. Cambridge: Cambridge University Press.

Nichter, Mark, and Margaret Lock, eds. 2002. *New horizons in medical anthropology.* London: Routledge.

Nowotny, Helga, Peter Scott, and Michael Gibbons. 2001. *Re-thinking science: Knowledge and the public in an age of uncertainty.* Cambridge: Polity.

Petryna, Adriana, Andrew Lakoff, and Arthur Kleinman, eds. 2006. *Global pharmaceuticals: Ethics, markets, practices.* Durham, NC: Duke University Press.

Rabeharisoa, Vololona. 2003. The struggle against neuromuscular diseases in France and the emergence of the "partnership model" of patient organisation. *Social Science & Medicine* 57:2127–36.

Rabeharisoa, Vololona, and Michel Callon. 2002. The involvement of patients' associations in research. *International Social Science Journal* 54, no. 1: 57–65.

———. 2004. Patients and scientists in French muscular dystrophy research. In *States of knowledge: The co-production of science and social order,* edited by Sheila Jasanoff, 142–60. London: Routledge.

Rabinow, Paul. 1992. Artificiality and enlightenment: From sociobiology to biosociality. In *Incorporations,* edited by J. Crary and S. Kwinter, 234–52. New York: Zone Books.

———. 1996. *Essays on the anthropology of reason.* Princeton, NJ: Princeton University Press.

Rapp, Rayna. 1999. *Testing women, testing the fetus: The social impact of amniocentesis in America.* London: Routledge.

Rapp, Rayna, and Faye Ginsburg. 2001. Enabling disability: Rewriting kinship, reimagining citizenship. *Public Culture* 13, no. 3: 533–56.

Rose, Nikolas. 2001. The politics of life itself. *Theory, Culture & Society* 18, no. 6: 1–30.

———. 2006. *The politics of life itself: Biomedicine, power and subjectivity in the twenty-first century.* Princeton, NJ: Princeton University Press.

Rose, Nikolas, and Carlos Novas. 2004. Biological citizenship. In *Global assemblages: Technology, politics, and ethics as anthropological problems,* edited by Aihwa Ong and Stephen Collier, 439–63. Oxford: Blackwell.

Sargent, Carolyn F., and Thomas M. Johnson, eds. 1996. *Medical anthropology: Contemporary theory and method,* rev. ed. Westport, CT: Praeger.

Schatzki, Theodore R., Karin Knorr Cetina, and Eike von Savigny, eds. 2001. *The practice turn in contemporary theory.* London: Routledge.

Scheper-Hughes, Nacy, and Loïc Wacquant, eds. 2003. *Commodifying bodies.* Theory, Culture & Society Series. London: Sage.

Schlich, Thomas, and Ulrich Troehler, eds. 2006. *The risks of medical innovation: Risk perception and assessment in historical context.* London: Routledge.

Strathern, Marilyn. 1992. *Reproducing the future: Essays on anthropology, kinship and the new reproductive technologies.* London: Routledge.

Sunder Rajan, Kaushik. 2006. *Biocapital: The constitution of post-genomic life.* Durham, NC: Duke University Press.

Thompson, Charis. 2005. *Making parents: The ontological choreography of reproductive technologies.* Cambridge, MA: MIT Press.

Timmermans, Stefan. 2005. Medicine, scientific. In *Science, technology, and society: An encyclopedia,* edited by Sal Restivo, 323–27. Oxford: Oxford University Press.

Timmermans, Stefan, and Marc Berg. 2003. *The gold standard: The challenge of evidence-based medicine and standardization in health care.* Philadelphia: Temple University Press.

Waldby, Catherine, and Robert Mitchell. 2006. *Tissue economies: Blood, organs, and cell lines in late capitalism.* Durham, NC: Duke University Press.

14   *Regula Valérie Burri and Joseph Dumit*

Young, Allan. 1995. *The harmony of illusions: Inventing posttraumatic stress disorder.* Princeton, NJ: Princeton University Press.
Zola, Irving K. 1972. Medicine as an institution of social control. *Sociological Review* 20, no. 4: 487–504.

Part I
Social and cultural studies of biomedicine

1 Medicalizing culture(s) or culturalizing medicine(s)

Stefan Beck

In December 2003, the Cyprus Bone Marrow Donor Registry—funded by a charity, the Karaiskakio Foundation—arranged a celebratory meeting of Cypriot donors and recipients of bone marrow grafts. A few days before Christmas, the invited persons, adults with their spouses and children accompanied by their parents, convened in a reception room of a big hotel in the capital, Nicosia. Two long tables were set—one labeled "donors," the other "recipients." As people trickled in, a father of a 10-year-old child who had successfully received a bone marrow graft in the beginning of the year excitedly approached the director of the registry and asked him who his son's benefactor was. However, the director, Pavlos Costeas, replied only, "At this table," indicating the "donors' desk" where already 10 people were sitting. Irritated, the father again asked who exactly the donor of the graft was that saved his son from dying of leukemia. Costeas repeated that this person was sitting at the "donors' desk" but firmly declared that he would not point him out. He explained that all donors present were united in the struggle to save the lives of leukemia sufferers. His rationale behind this policy is straightforward: Since only a fraction of all grafts provided by donors will actually be transplanted successfully, only some donors would be able to celebrate that they in fact had saved a life. What matters for Costeas, then, is the willingness to give and not the actual success of a transplantation; accordingly, the yearly celebration focuses on giving, not on saving.

In the present article, I will use the ethnographical account of this event (Badiou 2005: 173–83) as a focus to organize my argument.[1] The example I have chosen is somewhat distant from medical practices in the narrow sense; however, it will allow me to hint at some of the benefits and some of the problems that might occur when medicine is made into an object of anthropological scrutiny while using culture as a conceptual lens. This argument will be embedded in a rather sketchy critique of the specific disciplinary configurations in German-speaking countries, namely, the rich and highly problematic traditions of different anthropologies, a constellation most influential in defining disciplinary proximities and distances, research policies, and thought styles. It is argued that these intellectual traditions are not especially conducive for a research agenda that aims at analyzing recent biotechnological developments; therefore, some suggestions for amendments and disciplinary borrowings are made. It is claimed that a much broader account of medicine's direct and indirect effects on shaping professional as well as vernacular episteme and practices is vital. And it is suggested that medicine should take on the challenge to reflexively coproduce a vocabulary that allows others to come to terms, both socially and culturally, with its in(ter)ventions. Of course, this would necessitate a sustained collaboration with the social sciences and the humanities that surpasses fashionable interdisciplinary conversations and enters into a mode of in(ter)vention that coproduces instruments for cultural reflexivity.

MICRO EVENT: THE CREATION OF DIFFERENCE

New conceptual instruments for understanding novel entities, facts, and relationships brought into being through the application of biomedical technologies—of course—are not only wanted in the domain of transplantation medicine, though the obvious challenges for body images and the many social ambivalences immanent in donor–receiver relations provide a testing ground for the problem at hand. The guiding motivation of the director of the Cyprus Bone Marrow Donor Registry at these celebratory meetings is to protect the donors. As he told me, he had learned his lesson the hard way: Some years ago, he had to ask a donor to provide for a graft a second time because the first transplant had been rejected by the immune system of the receiver. The donor experienced this query as a devastating revelation. As he told Costeas, after having given the graft, he had lived for months in the elated conviction of having saved a life—an act, as he saw it, that had fundamentally changed his life. "But by asking me to give again," he said, "you have robbed me of my new identity and you have cast doubt on whether it will make sense to provide bone marrow again."

His experiences with the powerful effect of transformed self-perceptions of donors who "gave life" motivated Costeas to implement a policy of strict nondisclosure and anonymity in order to secure for all donors the conviction that they had contributed in a collective effort to save a life. As a result of this policy donors are removed from the registry to avoid a situation where they are asked to donate a second time. That this rule of strict, mutual anonymity between donors and recipients provides the framework for the intimate coming-together of donors and recipients in the Nicosia hotel a few days before Christmas might seem odd at first. It may appear particularly exotic if you compare this event to conventional practices in, for example, the United States, where meetings between donors and recipients are highly publicized, show-like happenings. There, survivors and their donors are meeting on the stages of big convention halls, falling into each other's arms under the applause of kin, friends, and a large audience. These events dramatize individual generosity that successfully has responded to individual suffering, followed by individual salvation of the sick, and resulting in individual pride on the part of the donor: a congregation of like-minded individuals is demonstrated. In contrast, the ritual developed by the Cyprus Bone Marrow Donor Registry celebrates donors as anonymous constituents of a collectivity. Salvation here is depersonalized, and altruism is collectivized.

It is noteworthy that Costeas shaped his policy in explicit contrast to the "American model" depicted before, a practice he had experienced during his education and work in an east coast university hospital. The creation of this highly ambivalent and even contradictory anonymous intimacy of the meetings has two purposes: first, to protect the donors from grief, namely, the realization that the recipient of the provided graft had died. However, what might even be more important in a small island society of merely 600,000 persons, where everybody is only some handshakes away from everybody else, is to reduce possible feelings of dependency or superiority between donors and recipients, a pressing problem, as will be demonstrated below.

A promising approach to investigate the implied problematics in the event might be to look at it by analyzing instances of social control at work on the micro level of interactions. And indeed, most anthropological studies in German-speaking countries, analyzing similar situations, are focusing on phenomena of domination and the transformation of "vernacular" practices working with the concept of medicalization. However, I suggest that this perspective—while affording a powerful tool—might not be the ideal candidate to analyze the heterogeneity of processes observable in this situation. Let me briefly explain why.

MEDICINE AS AGENT OF SOCIAL CONTROL: MEDICALIZATION AND ITS DISCONTENTS

Generally, medicalization signifies a process in which a medical frame or definition is applied to understand or manage a problem. Well-known examples are the emergence of professional groups such as physicians in the eighteenth century, the founding of medical institutions such as birthhouses in which poor women had to give birth under medically controlled conditions, or much more recently the emergence of new syndromes like attention deficit disorder that define a complex behavioral phenomenon as being caused by neurological states. Specifically, medicalization describes a process of social control in which phenomena, formerly understood to be nonmedical or nonproblematical, "become defined and treated as medical problems, usually in terms of illnesses or disorders" (Conrad 1992: 209). Early studies in medicalization processes in the late 1960s and early 1970s took their inspiration in part from Talcott Parsons (1951), who was "probably the first to conceptualize medicine as an institution of social control"

(Conrad 1992: 210). More often than not, medicalization is understood to be a linear process unfolding in modernity parallel and in part linked to secularization. To quote a famous definition from the early 1980s, it is a "process whereby more and more of everyday life has come under medical dominion, influence and supervision" (Zola 1983: 295). As such, medicalization is conceptualized as part of the disenchantment that is emblematic for modernization.

These processes can be observed on at least three levels: (1) on a conceptual level, for example, when a medical model is used to "order" or define a problem at hand; (2) on an institutional level, for example, when an organization or a political actor adopts a medical approach to treat a particular problem; (3) and, finally, on an interactional level "as part of the doctor-patient interaction" (Conrad 1992: 211).

Medicalization, understood from this perspective, is a multilevel controlling process (Nader 1997) that tends to unseat vernacular notions of health and disease and that substitutes popular customs in the domain of healing and curing with scientifically informed, therapeutic practices. In German-speaking cultural anthropology, this understanding of scientific medicine dominated discussions until recently. Of course, there are marked differences between two varieties of anthropological practice that emerged in German-speaking countries in the nineteenth century. It suffices to say that there is an institutionalized division between Volkskunde (folklore: the ethnology and anthropology of European cultures), on the one hand, and Völkerkunde (devoted to the anthropological study of non-European cultures), on the other. However, for the purpose of my argument, I can ignore most of the implications of this split here (Hauschild 1983). What is more important in the context of this line of reasoning is that both disciplines are still biased by the legacy of exotistic approaches to culture. As Beatrix Pfleiderer remarked in a review of ethnological and anthropological work in the domain of medicine, the disciplinary perspective was intricately shaped by studying "exotic," small-scale, nonindustrialized societies (Pfleiderer 1993: 365). Similarly, Volkskunde invested much of its energy in describing and recovering the exotic, the vernacular, and the suppressed in the margins of industrialized societies, to be found either in the distant past or in "distant" social strata, far removed from mainstream social life. While Völkerkunde specialized in describing Ethnomedizin (ethnomedicine), Volkskunde focused by and large on Volksmedizin (folk healing and traditional medicine under a well-defined historical perspective), analyzing those beliefs, concepts, and practices regarding disease and healing that were as far removed from scientific medicine as possible.

However, the 1970s and early 1980s saw a growing critique of these rather descriptive approaches that both tended to construct their objects of inquiry as bounded, essentialized entities, purged from influences of modernity. At the same time, German-speaking anthropologists gradually followed the international trend in their discipline to turn their professional attention on industrialized societies. One of the consequences of these critiques was a major reorientation of research programs in the 1980s. As Eberhard Wolff analyzed in a review of studies in cultural anthropology—that is, Völkerkunde and Volkskunde—this development brought about a growing interest in those problems, tensions, and conflicts that are produced by the clash of professional, scientific views on illness with the diversity of lay practices in the domain of health and suffering (Wolff 2001, 1998). For both Volkskunde as well as Völkerkunde, the concept of medicalization and the perspective of social control provided a compact and robust toolbox to analyze and critique historical as well as present developments in the domain of medicine. However, there are several problems with this concept—I will focus on two of them.

The first problem is that situations like those which I described at the beginning of this essay can only inadequately be analyzed using the model of medicalization. As, for example, Margaret Lock and Patricia Kaufert argue (1998), the main weakness of this concept is that it highlights the control and tends to render the contribution or the resistance of the controlled invisible. In this case, the Cyprus Bone Marrow Donor registry sets up meetings of donors and recipients that attempt to create an intimate anonymity between participants. The way they manage these meetings makes it evident that the organizers intend to define and control the social bond connecting the participants and the strong emotions that go with it—the pride and the elation of donors as well as the gratefulness and the joy of recipients. However, they are again and again beseeched by donors and recipients alike to disclose the identity of their respective counterparts. In this case, the object of social control as it is exercised by the registry is in itself a direct result of an adoption of medical options and technologies on the part of the participants.

This is to say that to become a donor or a recipient of a bone marrow graft is not simply to turn into an object of medical regimes. Instead, it means that donors and recipients of grafts are becoming enrolled in medical practices that afford a new subjectivity; for example, that of a proud bone marrow donor. These are practices that afford a new conception of one's own body—after all, live cells of the donor are living in the body of a fellow human—and practices that afford the competence to come to terms with novel technogenic kinship relations. The biomedical apparatus set in motion by the Cyprus Bone Marrow Donor Registry forms attitudes and self-confidence, delimits emotions, and commends self-restraint to produce histocompatible selves—an emergent, new form of life.

At the same time, these histocompatible selves draw on specifically Cypriot conceptions of community, solidarity, and altruism that make the Cypriot Bone Marrow Donor Registry one of the most successful biobanks worldwide: The Cyprus Registry is the fifth largest in Europe and the eleventh largest in the world. With more than 100,000 potential donors, it comprises more than 15 percent of the island population, compared to other registries in industrialized countries that comprise less than 2 percent of the population. Clearly, the success of the registry as well as the production of new forms of life that emerge in the epistemic space of histocompatibility (Müller-Wille & Rheinberger 2004), a space created by the amalgamation of biomedicine and cultural orientations, is only in part illuminated by the rather linear concept of medicalization, understood as a powerful form of social control. More refined models are called for that take into consideration the fact that controlling processes not only are historically and culturally contingent or necessarily unstable but also create new possibilities for disruption and the investment of meaning from below (Abel & Browner 1998).

However, there is a second, related set of possible problems created by the dominant culturalistic legacy in most German-language studies of medical issues. The tendency to take for granted a dichotomy between science and culture, on the one hand, supports simple models of medicalization. On the other hand, the appreciation of cultural pluralism creates the lingering relativism of medical pluralism.

MEDICINE AS CULTURE: ETHNOMEDICINES. HOWEVER, DOES SCIENCE HAVE CULTURE TOO?

Both problems are implied in the title of this essay. While the first plural—the cultures in "Medicalizing Culture(s) or Culturalizing Medicine(s)"—seems unproblematic, the second plural—the medicines—is somewhat precarious: If medicine is taken to refer to a scientific set of objectifying practices and facts, there is not much room for a colorful plurality. However, if the term *medicine* is not reserved for the Western-style medical system but instead conceived of in a very broad sense as organized health practices providing therapeutic choices for suffering individuals, then medicine "is so widespread around the globe that it is surely a universal in human organizations" (Kleinman 1995: 21). This assumed universality is reflected also in the term *ethnomedicine* that was coined in the tradition of the culture–science dichotomy to signify all "those beliefs and practices relating to disease which are the products of indigenous cultural development and are not derived from the conceptual framework of modern medicine" (Rubel & Hass 1996: 116). Understood in this broad sense, the plural "medicines" then appears largely unproblematic: It demarcates a research field that gives prominence to the conceptualizations of illness, its causes and cures, as well as the relationship between concepts of disease and cosmology in a specific group or society.

The pluralization of medicine here is highly compatible with the appreciation of cultural diversity past and present in mainstream social science in the late twentieth century. Medicines, as they are presented from this vantage point, are seen to pursue the identical aim—healing—since the beginning of time (Stengers 2000: 23). This identical aim, however, is pursued by highly diverse means and is accompanied by highly diverse understandings of disease. The main goal of a medical anthropology conceptualized along these lines would be to describe and understand this complexity and diversity in its dynamic cultural and social contexts.

Such studies have been particularly helpful in elucidating problems encountered in medical service provision for immigrant populations or in the implementation of development programs in non-Western countries. Anthropologists, for example, identified beliefs held by immigrant patients as a reason for noncompliance with medical advice. Anthropologists' contribution in this context has been to acknowledge alternative rationalities and practices. As a consequence, however, Western biomedicine also increasingly was analyzed along the lines of this model as just another cultural belief system and set of practices. But is it adequate to conceptualize biomedicine as the "ethnomedicine in which medical physicians are trained" (Rubel & Hass 1996: 116)?

Obviously, there is a conventional way to respond to this question: From the perspective of twentieth-century science, this view is completely unacceptable. Here, the concept of medical pluralism seems naïve in evoking either a dangerous relativism or even a belittling of charlatanism. This plural, then, is highly problematic, mainly because proper, scientific medicine—from the perspective of the sciences—is not like any other form of organized health practices. Instead, only those forms of health practices qualify as medicine that successfully pass the test of organized skepticism that science provides. Modern, scientific medicine, it follows, is a singularity produced—inter alia—by a long history of discriminating between quacks and physicians. As the historian of science Isabelle Stengers remarks, what allows the specific form of medicine called Western medicine or biomedicine "to lay claim to the title of science is not this or that medical innovation, but rather the way it diagnosed the power of the charlatan and explained the reasons to disqualify his power" (Stengers 2000: 24).

Scientific medicine, in this view, begins with the claim that not all cures are equally valid and effective and that not all medicines are equivalent. And scientific medicine proceeds by developing rigorous methods to differentiate between nonreproducible cures that depend on persons and circumstances, on the one hand, and, on the other hand cures, produced by verified procedures, that is, interventions that are statistically efficacious for everybody independent of local and personal contexts. And finally this *Idealtypus* of scientific medicine succeeds by refining and applying a materialistic understanding of human nature as physical to an ever-increasing number of behaviors and natural processes.

To analyze medicine as suggested here, namely, by analyzing its epistemic practices and regimes of truth, opens up an alternative to treating biomedicine as just another ethnomedicine. Instead, culturalizing medicine means to subject to cultural analysis the very epistemic practices that are shaping nosologies and etiologies, treatments and compliance, and patients and experts, no matter whether the medicine at hand is vernacular or scientific. And, of course, to inquire into the epistemic practices of medicine reveals without difficulty that the discrimination of scientific and "other" healing practices is hardly as clear-cut as the standard model of an ideal scientific medicine is implying. For example, the privileged instrument that is used to evaluate and assess interventions based on a scientific understanding of pathogenesis, the placebo test, creates a specific side effect: The test transforms a valuable feature of the living body, namely, to be responsive to hypnotizers, charlatans, and other nonreproducible, unexplainable individual processes, into a bad reason for recovery.

As the philosopher of science Isabelle Stengers puts it,

> When scientific medicine asks the public to share its values, it is asking the public to resist the temptation to be cured for "bad reasons.".... But why would ill people, who are interested only in their own cure, accept this distinction? (Stengers 2000: 24)

To safeguard this very distinction between good and bad reasons for recovery is what medicine is obsessed with: Precisely for the reason that it has to legitimate and defend its own position, it has to enlighten the public and fight against ethnomedical superstitions as well as detrimental attitudes.

The meetings organized by the Cyprus Bone Marrow Donor Registry are a case in point, where this commitment of biomedicine generates a comprehensive, paternalistic (in the best sense of the word) attitude toward their protégés. A culturalistic perspective might well correct the standard reproach that the biomedical system is inevitably characterized by a materialistic reductionism and decontextualism. Instead, as the meetings make clear, the officials of the registry see it as their obligation to educate actual and potential donors and recipients. In addition, they try to facilitate a congruous code of conduct and help to produce a *histocompatible subjectivity*. An analysis of these meetings, then, not only allows inquiries into embedding practices, the implementation of cosmopolitan biomedicine in a manner that is somehow sensitive to local culture. For anthropology, to take this analytic stance means to be concerned with medicine *in* culture. In addition, a culturalization of medicine also allows one to analyze medicine *as* culture. Under this perspective, orientations and practices of scientists and physicians are becoming visible as cultural. Consequently, scientists—for example—emerge as "moral entrepreneurs" who are deeply involved in cultural transformations.

However, analyzing medicine *as* culture also opens up a fresh perspective on knowledge practices and epistemic features in biomedicine, namely, the construction and fashioning of knowledge objects within science (Jordanova 1995; Amarasingham Rhodes 1996) or on the arrangements and mechanisms in biomedicine that shape what is known and how it is known (Toulmin 1976). In the following section, I will very briefly mention some recent approaches that analyze science and medicine under this perspective.

CULTURE(S) OF MEDICINE: EPISTEMIC CULTURE(S)

Arguably the two most influential studies for German-speaking social science that analyzed science as culture are Bruno Latour's *Laboratory Life* (Latour & Woolgar 1986) and Karin Knorr Cetina's *The Manufacture of Knowledge* (1981). Both studies, the first anthropological and the second sociological in their respective disciplinary backgrounds, used the theoretical framework as well as the methodological toolkit provided by cultural anthropology extensively to analyze the day-to-day practices and the minutiae of producing knowledge in laboratories. On the basis of long-term participant observation in molecular biology labs, both studies put forward that the groundwork of scientific creativity and originality was to be found in the seemingly boring and completely unspectacular routines of manipulating experimental settings. Instead of cognition, both studies proposed to focus on epistemic practices, and instead of analyzing individual acts of perception, both recommended analyzing social interactions and the collaborative fabrication of facts. From this perspective, science is characterized by practical, embodied thinking and problem solving, hardly distinct from everyday practices. Scientific facts, far from being pure mental objects, are interactively produced as results of material, experimental practices, biased observations, and contingent interpretations, based on established styles of thought. Social, technical, as well as cognitive norms are held as equally constitutive for science as the material and social environments scientists work in.

To study the machineries of knowledge construction and the epistemic cultures of science using this broad, culturalistic perspective reveals the fragmentation of contemporary medicine (Knorr Cetina 1999: 3) in exhibiting different architectures and empirical approaches in diverse specializations of medicine and the particular constructions of the referent in their respective epistemic settings. In other words, revealing the diversity of epistemic cultures disunifies medicine, opening up a comparative perspective that permits one to analyze practices in different medical systems. This differentiating perspective provides two immediate benefits: on the one hand, it directs attention to the interactions of medicines—in the plural—with diverse vernacular cultures—also in the plural. While science studies in the broad sense—that is history, sociology, and philosophy of science—concentrate on investigating scientific epistemic practices, cultural anthropologists studying science and medicine are encouraged by the traditions of their discipline to extend the scope of their studies also to the effects that scientific epistemic practices have on everyday cultures. On the other hand, this comparative perspective also functions as an antidote against the essentializing tendencies of many studies in German-speaking anthropology that used to treat biomedicine as a homogeneous entity.

MEDICINE'S CULTURAL PRODUCTIONS: NEW SOCIAL FORMS, EMERGENT SPHERES OF TRANSACTION

In the final section of this essay, attention shifts to the views of donors and receivers of bone marrow grafts and how they perceive the relations that are instigated by bone marrow transplantation. As already indicated, all receivers and life donors of organs and tissues share a like problem: How can the peculiar relationship between beneficiary and benefactor of a successful transplantation be conceptualized socially, culturally, and emotionally, and what are the social "models" participants can draw on to understand and tame this kind of odd intimate link to a person they do not know? I suggest that these donor–receiver relations represent a new type of biosocial relationship that is characterized by an anonymous intimacy and an intense entanglement with strangers that—due to its dependency on scientific knowledge—not only incorporates many ambivalences and uncertainties (Luhmann 1995) but also has the potential of disrupting other, more conventional social ties. However, this relationship also has the potential to engender new visions of the social, new visions of the self, and new visions of the biological afforded by this strange intimacy with strangers.

All Cypriot donors who took part in my research struggled how best to typify the exclusive relation that they—as they strongly felt—had created through the act of bone marrow donation to an unknown person. All of them thought about this person regularly, at least several times a week, and they were intensely concerned about the health of the patients. For most of them, donation was not the unproblematic closure of an often quite spontaneous decision to register, but it started a spiritual as well as a bodily entanglement that suddenly framed their life in an unexpected and profound way. The triviality of the medical procedure, the sampling of the graft—which requires a stimulation with a growth factor for four days, in some cases triggering mild, influenza-like symptoms, followed by a four-hour-long transfusion—is in stark disproportion to the felt social and spiritual effects. This sentiment is shared also by bone marrow recipients, who—while still perplexed that transplantation in the case of bone marrow transfer only means getting an injection with a "serum," a liquid containing stem cells that in the days after transplantation will drift into the bones and start producing blood cells—were very much aware of spiritual effects and rather unspecified social debts.

While the procedure of transplantation in the case of bone marrow seems trivial, it creates intimacies that are variously likened to "friendship," spiritual "kinship," or first-degree kinship. As a middle-aged businessman who gave bone marrow one year ago described his Other,

I feel that he is a piece/part of myself.... I see him as one of my most intimate persons. Now—if he is like my son or my brother—you cannot tell what makes the difference. You feel for all your family members in the same way.

For him, the relationship is even more intense—it is one of creation. As he told me,

> When I visited a monastery [some time after my donation], a nun told me, "His father gave him one life, you gave him a second one." I know that if there is not a matching donor, these patients cannot survive. I feel that I gave him life; it is something big what he got from me.

Similarly, a 45-year-old donor, feeling that she assisted her recipient to get "reborn," sees her Other as "a son." In contrast, a female donor in her late twenties is convinced that it would be improper to say that she had given life to the other person, but she is nevertheless convinced that the graft she gave "involved [her] whole physical life and [the] spiritual [as well]." Similarly, another recipient in her late teens would rather prefer to relate to her donor as a godparent, for many in Cyprus a still important, sacred form of spiritual relationship.

Here, as in all other conversations, the feeling of intimacy was clearly related not only to shared substance but also to the social form of donation and the supposed motifs of the donor: The grafts were given voluntarily and altruistically, meaning that no direct and explicit expectation to reciprocate was attached to them. Marilyn Strathern (1997: 300) has emphasized that according to Euro-American ideologies, or cosmologies (Sahlins 1996), the free will of all actors as well as the absence of self-interest are essential conditions of all intimate relationships, especially kinship relations. What has to be added, alas, is that according to these Euro-American concepts, intimacies also necessitate sustainable, mutual emotions (Swidler 2001; Zelizer 2005). What is at stake here becomes obvious in the statement of a young female donor: "I want to know how the [recipient] experienced it: How did he feel when he found out that there was a match, how he felt after the operation, and how he feels now?" Mutual emotional transparency as well as the ability to see and feel the presence and the bodily reactions of the Other are crucial for all respondents in order to "make the relation real"—as one female donor formulated: "To give him a warm hug. This is important because it makes [the relation] a whole. I will not live in a dream...when I see him, it is a reality."

However, due to the rules of anonymity, this strongly felt intensity of the "silent link" to the Other is frustratingly one-sided; the felt emotional connection is in marked contrast to the actual absence of any contact that would deserve the term *social*. All respondents felt very frustrated about this virtuality that they found difficult to cope with. In a way, they felt uncomfortable about their unshared emotions and felt embarrassed by their unreciprocated affections. As one young recipient expressed her grief about this enforced emotional solipsism,

> I have not met my donor yet and I have asked to meet him many times, I have cried for it, and [the physicians] don't tell me. I would like to meet him/her because I see him/her as part of my family. He/she is more than family.

All donors and most of the recipients were eagerly waiting for a sign of life of their Others, and they complained massively about the rules of strict anonymity that prevented them from meeting him or her. However, this anonymity was in most cases only an anonymity in principle: Somehow, all donors had gathered at least some intelligence about their recipients; for example, they had managed a glimpse into the papers during their trans-fusion, they knew about their receiver's nationality because they had suc-cessfully tricked their physicians into leaking information, or they used forensic imagination to extract information from the "thank-you cards" healed patients had finally sent after a year or two.

However, any accidental actualization of this virtual connection is likely to cause anxieties and deeply felt insecurities: In one exceptional case, the Cypriot recipient complained that the

> parents of my donor happen to know that I was the recipient and this bothers me. While I would like to forget about it, they constantly remind me of what happened. I don't know how they found out. But when I asked they told me, "You live in Cyprus." I think that this should not [happen].

In fact, the director of Karaiskakio Foundation takes every precaution so that what Pierre Bourdieu appropriately called "legitimate domination" will be avoided. According to Bourdieu, in acts of charity, where "the pos-sibility for an equivalent in return [is excluded]," there will be the likely effect that with "the very hope of an active reciprocity" also "the condition of possibility of genuine autonomy" is undermined. Here, the danger is imminent that lasting relations of dependency, legitimized by acts of altru-ism, will be created (Bourdieu 1997: 238ff.).

In the case of bone marrow donation, it is not only the irresolvable asymmetry between givers and receivers of gifts but also the—in this case, quite literal—personal extraction of the stem cells that is causing concern. As I have indicated before, donors gave away something they perceive as a crucial part of themselves: still living entities. In addition to the fact that gifts are perceived in consumerist culture as "extensions of the self" insofar as they are "expressions of personal sentiments" (Strathern 1997: 302), here the person of the giver sees him- or herself still inextricably attached to the extracorporeal cells: When the blood-building cells of the recipient are destroyed in preparation for the transplantation, in a way the *alter* of "alter ego" is removed and, with the transplantation at the latest, alter ego becomes—according to the views of most donors—ego, at least partially.

The same idea causes ruminations or at least insecure jokes on the part of recipients who wonder about the habits and lifestyle choices of their donors:

> I hope that he does not drink alcohol, smoke—I don't know whether physicians consider all these [things] before the extraction of bone marrow. I don't want to receive bone marrow from somebody who did such things, I never drank.

In part, of course, this young girl is afraid that the bone marrow she received might be of an inferior quality[2] because *her* donor was not health conscious enough. But here, as in other instances, there is also a marked horror of getting polluted or hybridized by what the Other did socially, what kind of character he has, and so on. This horror applies specifically also to those few Greek Cypriot recipients and laypersons who claim to feel reluctant to accept a graft from a Turkish donor; however, all respondents would happily provide a graft to a Turkish patient. This again points to the fact that all Greek Cypriot respondents are acutely aware of constellations of "legitimate domination"—through giving—or "inescapable submission"—through receiving. However, they never openly conceded that giving grafts would have the potential to fundamentally alter the constellation of the social field through amassing symbolic capital as a donor—or losing it as a recipient. The vocabulary provided by the medical profession, as well as the explicit vernacular theories of the "free gift," which is applied by all my respondents, clearly are not complex enough to cover these intricate social effects of practices of gift-giving.

It is vital, then, that instruments of disentanglement and purification are geared into action that somehow manage to establish a biosocial Green Line between donors and receivers so that they will not be tied together as dominant and dominated. What has to be purged—first—is the personal history of donors and the social context of their lives. Only as a filtrate, as pure and generic life, stem cells—programmed for an open future, without social history—are fit to be transferred. Secondly, any chance to reciprocate has to be excluded institutionally so that recipients are not to blame for not "giving back," a violation of the precept of *isotimia* (cf. Bourdieu 1997: 238), the affirmation that all participants are equal in honor. It is exactly this disentanglement that is achieved through the somewhat unfamiliar social arrangements at the Cypriot celebrations for donors and recipients: It provides instruments—discursive as well as pragmatic—with which to come to terms with culturally based expectations and apprehensions that do not prepare donors as well as recipients of bone marrow grafts to cope with the substantial links between strangers that have been brought into life by biomedicine.

MEDICINE AS CULTURE: ASSEMBLAGES, GLOCAL FORMS, EVENTS

It seems imperative that biomedicine takes on responsibility for the release of its strange entities and facts into culturally diverse environments. Of course, biomedical experts will be able to do so only in close collaboration with social science and the humanities: While most medical practitioners have accumulated—through praxis—dense circumstantial knowledges of those sociocultural environments that they act upon, this para-ethnography (Holmes & Marcus 2005) is more often than not prompted by failures in implementations of therapeutic regimes, suboptimal compliance, "mis-"understandings, and clandestine acts of resistance on the part of patients. It would seem beneficial to combine this dense knowledge based on reflexive praxis with deep knowledge based on ethnographical data and comparative accounts on sociocultural responses to the challenges posed by biomedicine. Wanted, then, are more sustained collaborations of medical practitioners and social scientists that inquire into the emergent cultural complexities and transformations in order to provide instruments for reflexivity, vocabularies to grasp the in(ter)ventions of biomedicine, and tools for understanding cosmological refractions generated by releasing facts and artifacts of biomedicine into diverse vernacular cultures.

These collaborations might offer added benefits for medicine and social science as well: On the one hand, anthropologists insist that the sociopolitical domain, namely, economic inequalities and global disparities in the allocation of medical resources in most cases, are more relevant in understanding differences regarding health practices than sociocultural differences between populations. One of the prominent representatives for this line of research cum activism in anthropology is Paul Farmer, who teaches anthropology at Harvard and directs a clinic in Haiti specializing in treating infectious diseases. Farmer proposes that anthropology should analyze the socioeconomic reasons that have made infectious diseases like the Ebola virus, tuberculosis, or HIV/AIDS "new epidemics." He is committed to developing a new research agenda for medical anthropology to inquire into the "multiple dynamics of health and human rights, on the health effects of war and political-economic disruption, [and] on the pathogenic effects of social inequalities, including racism, gender inequality, and the growing gap between rich and poor" (Farmer 2003: 241). And, in fact, recent studies in neuroendocrinology, in stress research or diabetes, for example, suggest that there are complex interdependencies between what is held to be social and biological. From this perspective, the anthropological focus on embodied minds provides an excellent starting point to begin collaborative work with medical researchers.

The second caution that anthropology offers against the overstraining of the culture concept comes from the global scope of the discipline that transcends interests in bounded cultures. Many recent studies do not define their research objectives in terms of culture at all, but instead choose infrastructures and frameworks of technologies on heterogeneous sociotechnical platforms as their objects. Peter Keating and Alberto Cambrosio, have introduced the notion of "biomedical platform" to refer to "material and discursive arrangements, or sets of instruments and programs, that, as timely constructs, coordinate [medical] practices and act as the bench upon which conventions concerning the biological or normal are connected with conventions concerning the medical or pathological" (Keating & Cambrosio 2000: 386). This concept, then, is able to correct some of the excesses of a "culturalistic reductionism," these all-too-idealistic constructivist approaches that tend to black-box techniques, instruments, and the materiality of scientific and medical practices.

Seen from this perspective, the meeting of donors and recipients of bone marrow transplants described in the beginning of this article can be analyzed as an event (Stengers 2000: 67ff.; Badiou 2005), where scientific practices, social norms, material structures, administrative routines, value systems, and legal regimes—that is, diverse regimes of truth production—are grouped together in a way that provides a basis for action and negotiation. This event is transformative in shaping subjectivities of participants as well as biomedical—material as well as discursive—practices. As such, it constitutes a prime target for anthropological curiosity.

NOTES

Acknowledgments. I appreciate the generous help of many colleagues and friends in the Cypriot health care sector, especially Pavlos Costeas, director of Karaiskakio Foundation, for the time he took in explaining the complexities—biological, political, administrative, bioethical, cultural, social, and psychological—that his work has to take into account. I thank his exceptional team for help in locating respondents, and Costas Constantinou, Intercollege, and Violetta Christophidou Anastasiadou, Makarios Hospital Nicosia, for enlightening discussions and sharing the material of the Cypriot part of the EU-funded research project "Challenges of Biomedicine (CoB)." I am grateful for the discussions with my colleagues Katrin Amelang (CoB subproject), Jörg Niewöhner (Collaboratory:Socialanthropology and LifeSciences, both Humboldt University at Berlin), and Gisela Welz (Frankfurt am Main) that helped in shaping the argument.

1. The ethnographic material was gathered in the fall of 2004 and the spring of 2005.
2. Strathern (1997: 301) suggests that anonymity secures that organs like "kidneys differ in physical condition rather than in social identity" (conceding, however, that "race" might be an uninvited guest in these reasonings). This is in contrast to nearly all the responding recipients, who—if only jokingly—referred to the imagined social identities of donors.

REFERENCES

Abel, Emily K., and C. H. Browner. 1998. Selective compliance with biomedical authority and the uses of experiential knowledge. In *Pragmatic women and body politics*, edited by Margaret Lock and Patricia A. Kaufert, 310–26. Cambridge: Cambridge University Press.

Amarasingham Rhodes, Lorna. 1996. Studying biomedicine as a cultural system. In *Contemporary theory and method*, rev. ed., edited by Carolyn F. Sargent and Thomas M. Johnson, 165–80. Westport, CT: Praeger.

Badiou, Alain. 2005. Being and event. New York: Continuum.

Bourdieu, Pierre. 1997. Marginalia—some additional notes on the gift. In *The logic of the gift: Toward an ethic of generosity*, edited by Alan D. Schrift, 231–41. New York: Routledge.

Conrad, Peter. 1992. Medicalization and social control. *Annual Review of Sociology* 18: 209–32.

Farmer, Paul. 2003. *Pathologies of power: Health, human rights, and the war on the poor*, foreword by Amartya Sen. Berkeley: University of California Press.

Hauschild, Thomas. 1983. Zur Einführung—Formen Europäischer Ethnologie. In *Europäische Ethnologie. Theorie- und Methodendiskussion aus ethnologischer und volkskundlicher Sicht*, edited by Heide Nixdorf and Thomas Hauschild, 11–26. Berlin: Reimer.

Holmes, Douglas and George E. Marcus. 2005. Cultures of Expertise and the Management of Globalization: Toward the Re-functioning of Ethnography. In *Global Assemblages. Technology, Politics, and Ethics as Anthropological Problems*, edited by Aihwa Ong and Stephen J. Collier. 235–52. Oxford: Blackwell.

Jordanova, Ludmilla. 1995. The social construction of medical knowledge. *Social History of Medicine* 3:361–82.

Keating, Peter, and Alberto Cambrosio. 2000. Biomedical platforms. *Configurations* 8:337–87.

Kleinman, Arthur. 1995. *Writing at the margin: Discourse between anthropology and medicine*. Berkeley: University of California Press.

Knorr Cetina, Karin. 1981. *The manufacture of knowledge: An essay on the constructivist and contextual nature of science*. Oxford: Pergamon.

———. 1999. *Epistemic cultures: How the sciences make knowledge*. Cambridge, MA: Harvard University Press.

Lock, Margaret, and Patricia A. Kaufert. 1998. Introduction. In *Pragmatic women and body politics*, edited by Margaret Lock and Patricia A. Kaufert, 1–27. Cambridge: Cambridge University Press.

Latour, Bruno, and Steve Woolgar. 1986. *Laboratory life: The construction of scientific facts*. Princeton, NJ: Princeton University Press.

Luhmann, Niklas. 1995. Die Soziologie des Wissens: Probleme ihrer theoretischen Konstruktion. In *Gesellschaftsstruktur und Semantik. Studien zur Wissenssoziologie der modernen Gesellschaft*, vol. 4, edited by Niklas Luhmann, 151–80. Frankfurt am Main: Suhrkamp.

Müller-Wille, Staffan, and Hans Jörg Rheinberger. 2004. *Heredity: The production of an epistemic space*. Preprint no. 276. Berlin: MPI für Wissenschaftsgeschichte.

Nader, Laura. 1997. Controlling processes. Tracing the dynamic components of power. *Current Anthropology* 38, no. 5: 711–37.

Parsons, Talcott. 1951. *The social system*. New York: Free Press.

Pfleiderer, Beatrix. 1993. Medizinanthropologie: Herkunft, Aufgaben und Ziele. In *Handbuch der Ethnologie*, edited by Thomas Schweizer, Margarete Schweizer, and Waltraud Kokot, 345–74. Berlin: Werner Reimer.

Rubel, Arthur J., and Michael R. Hass. 1996. Ethnomedicine. In *Contemporary theory and method*, rev. ed., edited by Carolyn F. Sargent and Thomas M. Johnson, 113–30. Westport, CT: Praeger.

Sahlins, Marshall. 1996. The sadness of sweetness: The native anthropology of Western cosmology. *Current Anthropology* 37, no. 3: 395–428.

Stengers, Isabelle. 2000. *The invention of modern science*, Theory Out of Bounds series, vol. 19. Minneapolis: University of Minnesota Press.

Strathern, Marilyn. 1997. Partners and consumers: Making relations visible. In *The logic of the gift: Toward an ethic of generosity*, edited by Alan D. Schrift, 292–311. New York: Routledge.

Swidler, Anne. 2001. *Talk of love: How culture matters*. Chicago: University of Chicago Press.

Toulmin, Stephen. 1976. On the nature of the physician's understanding. *Journal of Medicine and Philosophy* 1, no. 1: 32–50.

Wolff, Eberhard. 1998. "Volksmedizin"—Abschied auf Raten. Vom definitorischen zum heuristischen Begriffsverständnis. *Zeitschrift für Volkskunde* 94, no. 2: 233–57.

———. 2001. Volkskundliche Gesundheitsforschung, Medikalkultur- und "Volksmedizin"-Forschung. In *Grundriß der Volkskunde. Einführung in die Forschungsfelder der Europäischen Ethnologie*, edited by Rolf W. Brednich (3rd, enlarged ed.), 617–35. Berlin: Dietrich Reimer Verlag.

Zelizer, Viviana A. 2005. *The purchase of intimacy*. Princeton, NJ: Princeton University Press.

Zola, Irving K. 1983. *Socio-medical inquiries: Recollections, reflections and reconsiderations*. Philadelphia: Temple University Press.

2 Metaphors of medicine and the culture of healing
Historical perspectives

Jakob Tanner

This essay is intended to provide a historical perspective on the role of metaphors in medicine and the relevance of various cultures of healing. This last notion is itself prone to metaphorical transfers, because "healing" not only means the recovery from a disease or injury but also connotes emphatic concepts of health, fortune, salvation, and redemption. Words and images are mobilized to generate discourses of physical and mental perfection and to construct a utopia of eternal happiness. These imaginings take us far beyond a realistic assessment of the capacities and future potentials of modern medicine, and the more opaque such expectations are, the more seductive metaphorical operations become.

Since medical systems and practices are very complex and are subject to many contradictory influences and divergent requirements, their description shows a strong inclination to rely upon metaphorical operations. This attitude has been contested by authors like Susan Sontag, who wrote in her illuminating essay "Illness as Metaphor," "My point is that illness is not a metaphor, and that the most truthful way of regarding illness—and the healthiest way of being ill—is one most purified of, most resistant to, metaphoric thinking" (Sontag 1979: 3). Also, this "truthful way" is not completely free of metaphors, but it is based on a serious will to restrict their power on the understanding of what an illness is.

Before addressing how metaphorical operations and discursive dispositives have worked in the past and have been approached in historical studies of science and medicine, I will first explore what could be understood as a historical perspective on biomedicine as culture, and I will raise crucial questions of current interest for the historical understanding of biomedicine as a field of cultural practice.

CONTRADICTIONS AND COMPLEXITY IN THE HISTORY OF MEDICINE

The understanding of illness and medicine depends on significantly changing and different sociocultural and socioeconomic contexts. The problem is how to define the topic in a "historical perspective." Such a perspective can be developed—according to the ambivalence of the word *history*—in a very different way. "History" refers to both the academic discipline and the past, which can be described in a variety of ways. History means writing about the past with scientifically approved and methodologically sound procedures—and history designates the past as an inexhaustible resource for the creation of historical interpretations. The modern notion of history is based on the integration of the two meanings: The past is definitely gone, without, however, surrendering its intriguing hold on contemporary efforts at self-understanding made by individuals, social groups, and entire societies. The past is thus paradoxically absent and present at the same time. It is the task of the discipline of history, as a scientific practice, to propose an interpretation of the past: an account of the way bygone eras can be represented in the present (Koselleck 1971). It is an open question whether a historical perspective on (bio-)medical practices must render an account of all the concepts, theories, and approaches used in history today, or whether it should aim at demonstrating how history has treated medicine as a subject of analysis in earlier periods. Not claiming any completeness but rather driven by particular cases and aspects, I will deploy both approaches.[1]

For a long time, the history of medicine has been embedded in a narrative of progress, which contrasted the orthodoxy of science-based medicine and medical practice with various forms of folk medicine or quackery. This view was legitimized by the enormous progress in the practice of medicine, especially in the field of surgery and regarding the pharmaceutical-based treatments, during the nineteenth and twentieth centuries. Basically, modern Western medicine was considered to be the outcome of a systematic replacement of superstition by science. Although historians had always been aware that a great variety of stories of illness and healing persisted in every period, they often judged the validity of such popular interpretations in the light of modern biomedicine and stigmatized alternative solutions as irrational, fraudulent, or even dangerous. Every assessment of medical practices was rooted in a deep belief in scientific knowledge, technology-based procedures, and rational methods.

Surprisingly, this view was not challenged by social historians but, rather, in the somewhat specialized field of medical history as well as in science and technology studies (STS). Dissenting voices could be heard as early as 1935, when Ludwik Fleck in his famous study on the "Genesis and Development of a Scientific Fact" stated that modern medicine is not and cannot be a scientific discipline based in one single paradigm (Fleck 1979). Fleck pointed out that the multifaceted, complex nature of medical practice entailed that doctors were always having to cope with situations in which urgent action was required without having a clear idea of the relevant theoretical assumptions. There is a great divide between the knowledge of a situation and the expertise required to deal with it. Medical practices have a tacit dimension: They are rooted in the human body, in implicit skills, which cannot be spelled out in a manner appropriate to scientific theory. Michael Polanyi spelled out such a theory of the "tacit dimension" in the 1950s and 1960s (Polanyi 1958/1998, 1967). Thus, science is often used to veil the implicit dimension of medical agency. Among physicians, such a resistance to the theoretical illumination of medical practice is widespread. As Arthur Kleinman puts it, "Clinicians tend to be simplistic about clinical practice. Their tendency toward positivistic scientism and atheoretical pragmatism discourages attempts to understand illness and care as embedded in the social and cultural world" (Kleinman 1980: xii).

Another considerable influence on the conceptualization of "Western medicine" in history has come from cultural anthropology, mostly from researchers in the tradition of Franz Boas who have abandoned the Euro- and ethnocentrisms typical of one-dimensional occidental rationalism and universalism. The attempt to make sense of cultural differences introduces what might be called (with Donald Davidson) a "principle of charity" into intercultural communication and translation processes (Davidson 2001). This principle tries to make sense out of cultural differences and allows optimizing agreement between ourselves and those we interpret. More to the point, it permits a new understanding of the hidden logic and cultural significance of what seem at first to be unfamiliar medical practices. By the end of the 1950s, a growing concern about the short-sighted philosophical assumptions of biomedical concepts emerged. When Erwin H. Ackerknecht published his *Short History of Psychiatry* in 1958, he dedicated the book to the anthropologist Ruth Benedict; in an "anthropological introductory remark," he wrote,

> Let's assume that the occurrence and the definition of mental disorders is related to social conditions. Thus we must also assume that mental disorders vary in terms of frequency and form from tribe to tribe, from culture to culture, from civilization to civilization. This is in fact the case. (Ackerknecht 1958/1985: 5)[2]

This view was supported by a growing number of authors, and attracted attention to researchers in the field of history as well. Based on this argument, Arthur Kleinman noted in the *Encyclopedia of the History of Medicine* (published in 1993), "Biomedicine is, like all forms of medicine, both the social historical child of a particular world with its particular pattern of time and an institution that over time develops its own unique form and trajectory" (Kleinman 1993: 22). This trajectory reflects, after all, "the Western tradition's idea of progress" and is bound to a "radically reductionistic and positivistic value orientation" with "dehumanizing" effects (20, 18).

In the postwar period, philosophers were also starting to reexamine medical practices and the patient–doctor relationship.[3] In 1958, Karl Jaspers, who had himself been a physician before becoming a psychotherapist and then a philosopher, describes in *The Medical Practitioner in the Technical Age* how patients who seek constant treatment make impossible claims on their doctors, thereby enforcing therapies which are in no way rationally effective. Jaspers quotes a pharmacist as saying, "We have a dozen effective cures; the rest is a product of the anxiety of the patient and the interests of the industry" (Jaspers 1958/1986: 10).[4] Thus emotions like fear and hope, producing perhaps placebo effects which cannot be explained in a coherent way, must be taken into account as decisive factors affecting the medical system.

This view becomes even more persuasive when alternative or complementary medical practices turn out to be more and more popular not only in marginal sectors of modern societies but also in the citadels of medical science and technology in the industrialized nations. These approaches, which are also labeled holistic or integrative, are based in therapeutic practices which are not subjected to the standard proofs of efficacy common in science-based biomedicine; nonetheless, they prove to be both productive and profitable in many situations. Health insurance companies increasingly acknowledge such approaches since they are aware of the economic potential of placebo effects and phantom risks (Foster et al. 1993; Spiro 1998).

In this new context, traditional historiography, which for a long time has been committed to the role of an apologist for modern biomedicine, has lost a great deal of its former plausibility. New approaches to the history of medicine overcame the artificial separation between esoteric scientific knowledge and popular belief systems, thereby advancing the understanding of medicine as a cultural and social phenomenon. Social historians like Thomas McKeown (1976/1979) have shown that the betterment of health conditions and the prolongation of life expectancy are mostly due to social improvements in nutrition, housing, and clothing as well as in the formation of human capital. They have criticized the reductionist perception of the human body as a mechanical device or a "human motor" which can be controlled and regulated by biomedical interventions. In the 1970s, McKeown and Archibald L. Cochrane were two of the most influential voices in criticizing the dominance of biomedical thinking. A bibliometric study of the references to McKeown's *The Role of Medicine* (1976/1979) and Cochrane's *Effectiveness and Efficiency* (1972) shows how their ideas have been disseminated (Alvarez-Dardet & Ruiz 1993). It suggests that these two books have been important in stimulating new knowledge and in linking history with other disciplines. It is quite obvious that the main problems identified by McKeown and Cochrane—namely, the relatively small impact of clinical medicine on health outcomes and the poor use of scientific methods in clinical practice—are still with us and present in current debates on what is called an "evidence-based medicine."

In her study *Medicine as Culture* (1994/2003), Deborah Lupton elaborates on the cultural analysis of the paradoxes and contradictions of modern medicine. Western societies, she writes, are today "characterized by people's increasing disillusionment with scientific medicine." Access to medical care is widely regarded as a social good and the inalienable right of every person. Beyond that, medical views on health and the body dominate public discourse and private discussions, and faith in medicine has become a creed (Lupton 1994/2003: 1; see also Le Fanu 1999). On the one hand, Lupton underlines, dependence on biomedicine as the provider of answers to social as well as medical problems remains high, while, on the other hand, "doctors are criticized for abusing their medical power by controlling or oppressing their patients, for malpractice and indulging in avarice" (Lupton 1994/2003: 1). Lupton concludes

> that in Western societies, as in all other societies, issues of health, illness, disease and death are inextricably interlinked with social processes; that is, the biological dimensions...cannot easily be extricated from the socio-cultural settings in which they are known and experienced. (173)

SEMIOTICS, TECHNOLOGIES, PRACTICES

Such premises have taken on increasing importance in controversies among historians. Currently, four aspects are of particular interest for the historical understanding of biomedicine as culture; that is, the analysis of the interrelationship between cultural change and shifts in medical approaches.

Firstly, medicine as a cultural practice is related to both power and knowledge. Michel Foucault's concepts of biopolitics and biopower refer to judicial power and disciplinary techniques and mark the introduction of the notion of a social body as the object of government (e.g., Foucault 1980). Biopolitics is concerned with population as a political and scientific issue, as a biological substrate for the exercise of power in a preventive fashion. Its legitimacy stems from "the power to make live," that is, from its promise to optimize life chances. The government of biopower works through the management and regulative mechanisms that allow controlling probabilistic risks and unpredictable phenomena on a local as well as on a global scale (Foucault 2004a, 2004b). Apparently, medicine is one of the sensitive fields for the implementation of such strategies in a population. This can be shown by focusing on the specialization and state-supported professionalization of a growing group of medical experts.

Secondly, the definition and classification of diseases are based on language and intertwined with cognitive pattern recognition and template matching. As Roland Barthes (1988) and others have shown, modern semiotics was developed in a science-based medicine, where it derives from the necessity to integrate diverse indications, polysemic expressions, and often contradicting signs into a coherent framework of denotations for diseases. This way, etiology (classification by cause) and pathogenesis (classification according to the mechanism in which agents cause diseases) become possible. An alternative system—nosology—involves the difficulty that many diseases affect multiple organs. In fact, diagnostic terms are often just names for either symptoms or whole sets of symptoms, that is, syndromes. This opens the insight that diseases are culturally constructed; they are thus malleable entities and as such comparable to conceptions of health.

This strengthens thirdly the proposition that the definition of diseases and clinical categories are the outcomes of different cultures. There is no such thing as a "true" etiology or nosology for the human body in general, but a whole variety of different perceptions and classifications. Medical experts, who are interested in medical phenomena beyond their own cultural horizon, are permanently lost in translation. Without cross-cultural analyses and international comparisons in the framework of an entangled history, or a shared history, there would be no appropriate understanding of gender- and class-related "medical systems" and therapeutic practices in different societies.

Fourthly, it is important to see how the development of new (visual) diagnostic methods and the innovation of therapeutic trajectories have transformed not only etiological explanations and nosographical classifications but also the subjective experience of health and illness. Private perceptions of bodily sensations and the state of mind are not isolated from dominant modes of interpretation; they are also affected by the materiality of media and technical tools, which interfere in self-perception and auto-understanding of individuals and social groups. Technically mediated images are one example which shifts the boundary of what can be seen by the eye into the dark zones of the body. Functional neuroimaging, MRI in general, and visual representations of the human embryo are constructions based on highly sophisticated methods of data gathering, mathematical models, and efficient, computer-driven information processing (cf. Heintz & Huber 2001; Burri 2001; Duden 1994; Gugerli & Orland 2002).

Many of the highly sophisticated studies of methods in molecular medicine, functional tissue engineering, tissue remodeling and reparative medicine, and human cell culture protocols still rely on a concept of culture that frames culture as the successful technical control of natural phenomena, and aims to develop entirely new strategies of healing and improving the human body. Recent approaches in the social studies of science, however, emphasize that the common use of the concept of culture contains interesting implications because "culture," as in the breeding of bacteria and other microbes or cells in an artificial environment by means of laboratory techniques, constitutes a culture–nature hybrid (Latour 1993; Goodman et al. 2003). It represents the application of scientific knowledge and experimental skills to a decontextualized and controlled nature. Nature is transformed into a resource for therapeutic strategies to "repair" or improve individual human bodies in line with the main values of a postmodern society: beauty, youth, and longevity. The notion of "biosociology" (in criticizing the concept of "sociobiology"), as introduced by Paul Rabinow

(1996) in order to analyze the sociocultural shaping of human-engineering technologies, is of particular interest in this regard.

In addition to this biotechnical approach, the notion of "culture" (related to medicine) is also used when referring to traditional or alternative forms of healing. Australian Aborigines and the "ritual healing in Navajo society," for example, are presented as being profoundly different from Western culture and medicine in their symbolic operations and social logics (e.g., Hunter 1993; Csordas 2000). This is also valid for historical studies on the "folk medicine" or alternative and complementary healing practices in industrial societies (e.g., Jütte 1998). Thus, in a strange juxtaposition, the concept of "culture" is used in relation to both the most advanced technoscientific practices, and healing practices drawing on other than biomedical expertise.

DISCOURSIVE DISPOSITIVES AND METAPHORICAL OPERATIONS

Explorations in the borderland shared by anthropology, medicine, and psychiatry have provided new insights into the changing contexts in which physicians and healers are working. The "linguistic turn" in the humanities in the 1980s (cf. Hunt 1989; Barberi 2000; Trabant 2005) has enhanced the sensibility of transdisciplinary research for metaphoric operations and discursive "dispositives" (cf. Foucault 1991). This perspective includes not only medical practices but also the self-definition of patients—the so-called patient's view. It also goes along with healing processes and the stability of social structures and with a confidence in shared mental models and in the power of phantasms, especially those linked with the "body as a battlefield" which is exposed to invasions of invisible enemies and has therefore to be defended (Vigarello 1988). Mythologies also play an important role. Roland Barthes's definition has not lost any of its explanatory power today:

> Myth is constituted by the loss of the historical quality of things: in it, things lose the memory of how they were made. The world enters language in a dialectical relation between activities, between human actions; it comes out of myth as a harmonious display of essence. (Barthes 1964: 130)

Furthermore, as Barthes has also shown, both the language and the visual representations of medicine have shaped expectations in society regarding the maintenance of health and healing from diseases.

Both myth and fantasy deploy metaphorical operations (Fracchia & Lewontin 2005). In the very beginnings of Western medicine, in Greece, important metaphors for the unity and harmony of the body were adapted from the arts and from technology. Thus, scientific explanations have been in the grip of fantasies and diseases, and overlaid with mystifications (Sontag 1979: 87). A significantly innovative period took place during the rise of microbiology and bacteriology in the nineteenth century. These disciplines gave modern hygiene and medicine a growing reputation; since the 1880s, new theories and medications have seemed to promise a rebirth of modern scientific medicine, thereby putting an end to the "therapeutic nihilism" of the decades before. In her illuminating book *Membranes: Metaphors of Invasion in Nineteenth-Century Literature, Science, and Politics*, Laura Otis notes that "both cells and bacteria became known as well-defined, independent entities." The cell as the locus of disease and the microbe as its cause initiated a shift of attention from physical environments toward the people who inhabit them. "This change in perspective indicates an increasing tendency to conceive of life and disease in terms of units with distinct boundaries." This image corresponds closely with the bourgeois model— or ideal—of the free, responsible, and "self-contained" individual, which is also a guarantee of good health (Otis 1999: 8ff.).

Imperial Germany affords a good example of just how closely scientific and political semantics have been interrelated. Both bacteriology and politics have relied upon a powerful image of invisible, inferior, but potent enemies. Along with a mutual interchange of metaphors and vocabularies, bacteriological hygiene has been thought to provide solutions to social problems. The public was electrified by the spectacular proofs of Robert Koch and Louis Pasteur, who became scientific celebrities in the early 1880s. Medical metaphors were incorporated in the political language of the time (Gradmann 2000). Together with popular authors, famous researchers like Robert Koch launched the "glorious war of destruction on all of the micro-riffraff." In 1882, Koch described bacteria as mischievous agents, capable of interfering in wars in the form of the weapon of epidemics. He proposed the following picture:

> [Bacteria] creep around and live off the marrow of the army even in times of peace; but once the torch of war blazes, and then they creep out from their crevices, raise their heads to a colossal height, and destroy everything that is in the way. Proud armies have often been decimated, even destroyed, by epidemics; wars and thus the fate of peoples have been decided by them. (Robert Koch, quoted in Gradmann 2000: 25)

This language of war and fear, of attack and defense, which uses the human body as a battlefield, was enormously resistant over time and survived all institutional changes. Today, it is reactivated in a new context, which uses anxieties and fears of broad strata of the population.

In his already mentioned essay "The Medical Practitioner in the Technical Age" from 1958, Karl Jaspers notes that the modern citizen has transformed his transcendent faith into a mundane belief in the problem-solving capacity of technical systems and scientific practices. It is the rise of a "technological society," Jaspers claims, which has deprived humans of their deep sense of immortality, and they have thus become objects of technical health maintenance and medical interventions. Nevertheless, the modern subject has not lost his or her yearning for a spiritual dimension. Against this background, the emergence of psychosomatics can be interpreted as the joint effect of an epoch devoid of transcendental confidence and, at the same time, desperately seeking personal salvation and redemption.

This dilemma has been accentuated by the fact that promising new technologies like genetics, reproductive medicine, or organ transplantation have replaced the notion of "normal health" with that of "peak performance" (Rothman & Rothman 2003). Such an optimal state can be achieved only through a technomedical reshaping of the body, paralleled by a refashioning of the self. As a result, the century-old tension between high-flying expectations and promises and the realization that the power of both physicians and medical drugs remains limited and precarious has been intensified. In modern societies, which are characterized by persisting and even increasing social inequalities and new forms of exclusion, this problem is also linked to the future of the welfare state and the general access to health care and medical treatment. This raises the question of whether the mythopoetic anticipation of a bright future will foster identification with modern medical technologies or result in a frustrating disappointment about ongoing technological advances and empty promises. The most persuasive hypothesis suggests that this ambivalence will never disappear, and will therefore continue to be relevant in the future.

NOTES

1. Classical accounts of the history of medicine are Ackerknecht (1992) and Lock (2001).
2. This citation is from the preamble of the 1957 edition.
3. For an overview, see Rosenberg (1979).
4. My translation. See also Krimsky (2003) and Angell (2004).

REFERENCES

Ackerknecht, Erwin H. 1958/1985. *Kurze Geschichte der Psychiatrie.* Stuttgart: Ferdinand Enke Verlag.
——. 1992. *Geschichte der Medizin.* Stuttgart: Enke.
Alvarez-Dardet, C., and M. T. Ruiz. 1993. Thomas McKeown and Archibald Cochrane: A journey through the diffusion of their ideas. *British Medical Journal* 306, no. 6687 (May 8): 1252–54.
Angell, Marcia. 2004. *The truth about the drug companies: How they deceive us and what to do about it.* New York: Random House.
Barberi, Alessandro. 2000. *Clio verwunde(r)t. Hayden White, Carlo Ginzburg und das Sprachproblem der Geschichte.* Vienna: Turia + Kant.

44 Jakob Tanner

Barthes, Roland. 1964. *Mythen des Alltags.* Frankfurt am Main: Suhrkamp.
————. 1988. *Das semiologische Abenteuer.* Frankfurt am Main: Suhrkamp.
Burri, Regula Valérie. 2001. Doing images: Zur soziotechnischen Fabrikation visueller Erkenntnis in der Medizin. In *Mit dem Auge denken: Strategien der Sichtbarmachung in wissenschaftlichen und virtuellen Welten,* edited by Bettina Heintz and Joerg Huber, 277–303. Zürich: Springer, Edition Voldemeer.
Cochrane, Archibald Leman. 1972. *Effectiveness and efficiency: Random reflections on health services.* London: Nuffield Provincial Hospitals Trust.
Csordas, Thomas J., guest ed. 2000. Ritual healing in Navajo society. *Medical Anthropology Quarterly* 14, no. 4 (special issue).
Davidson, Donald. 2001. *Inquiries into truth and interpretation.* Oxford: Oxford University Press.
Duden, Barbara. 1994. *Der Frauenleib als öffentlicher Ort: vom Missbrauch des Begriffs Leben.* München: Deutscher Taschenbuch-Verlag.
Fleck, Ludwik. 1979. *Genesis and development of a scientific fact,* edited by Thaddeus J. Trenn and Robert K. Merton, foreword by Thomas S. Kuhn. Chicago: University of Chicago Press.
Foster, Kenneth R., David E. Bernstein, and Peter W. Huber, eds. 1993. *Phantom risk: Scientific inference and the law.* Cambridge, MA: MIT Press.
Foucault, Michel. 1980. *Power/knowledge: Selected interviews and other writings, 1972–1977.* New York: Pantheon.
————. 1991. *Der Wille zum Wissen, Sexualität und Wahrheit* Bd. 1. Frankfurt am Main: Suhrkamp.
————. 2004a. *Naissance de la biopolitique. Cours au Collège de France, 1978–1979.* Paris: Gallimard Seuil.
————. 2004b. *Sécurité, Territoire, Population. Cours au Collège de France, 1977–1978.* Paris: Gallimard Seuil.
Fracchia, Joseph, and R. C. Lewontin. 2005. The price of metaphor. *History and Theory. Studies in the Philosophy of History* 44, no. 1: 14–29.
Goodman, Alan H., Deborah Heath, and M. Susan Lindee, eds. 2003. *Genetic nature/culture: Anthropology and science beyond the two-culture divide.* Berkeley: University of California Press.
Gradmann, Christoph. 2000. Invisible enemies. *Science in Context* 13, no. 1: 9–30.
Gugerli, David, and Barbara Orland, eds. 2002. *Ganz normale Bilder. Historische Beiträge zur visuellen Herstellung von Selbstverständlichkeit.* Zürich: Chronos.
Heintz, Bettina, and Joerg Huber, eds. 2001. *Mit dem Auge denken: Strategien der Sichtbarmachung in wissenschaftlichen und virtuellen Welten.* Zürich: Springer, Edition Voldemeer.
Hunt, Lynn, ed. 1989. *The new cultural history.* Berkeley: University of California Press.
Hunter, Ernest. 1993. *Aboriginal health and history: Power and prejudice in remote Australia.* Cambridge: Cambridge University Press.
Jaspers, Karl. 1958/1986. *Der Arzt im technischen Zeitalter.* München: Springer.
Jütte, Robert, et al., eds. 1998. *Culture, knowledge and healing: Historical perspectives of homeopathic medicine in Europe and North America.* Sheffield, UK: EAHMH.
Kleinman, Arthur. 1980. *Patients and healers in the context of culture: An exploration of the borderland between anthropology, medicine, and psychiatry.* Berkeley: University of California Press.
————. 1993. What is specific to Western medicine. In *Encyclopedia of the history of medicine,* edited by W. F. Bynum and Roy Porter. New York: Routledge.

Koselleck, Reinhart. 1971. Wozu noch Historie? *Historische Zeitschrift* 212, no. 1: 1–18.

Krimsky, Sheldon. 2003. *Science in the private interest: Has the lure of profits corrupted biomedical research?* Lanham, MD: Rowman & Littlefield.

Latour, Bruno. 1993. *We have never been modern.* Cambridge, MA: Harvard University Press.

Le Fanu, James. 1999. *The rise and fall of modern medicine.* London: Little, Brown.

Lock, Stephen, ed. 2001. *The Oxford illustrated companion to medicine.* Oxford: Oxford University Press.

Lupton, Deborah. 1994/2003. *Medicine as culture: Illness, disease and the body in Western societies*, 2nd ed. London: Sage.

McKeown, Thomas. 1976/1979. *The role of medicine: Dream, mirage or nemesis?* Oxford: Blackwell.

Otis, Laura. 1999. *Membranes: Metaphors of invasion in nineteenth-century literature, science, and politics.* Baltimore: John Hopkins University Press.

Polanyi, Michael. 1958/1998. *Personal knowledge: Towards a post-critical philosophy.* London: Routledge.

———. 1967. *The tacit dimension.* London: Anchor.

Rabinow, Paul. 1996. *Essays on the anthropology of reason.* Princeton, NJ: Princeton University Press.

Rosenberg, Charles. 1979. The therapeutic revolution: Medicine, meaning, and social change in nineteenth-century America. In *The therapeutic revolution: Essays in the social history of American medicine*, edited by Charles Rosenberg and Morris Vogel. Philadelphia: University of Pennsylvania Press.

Rothman, Sheila M., and David J. Rothman. 2003. *The pursuit of perfection: The promise and perils of medical enhancement.* New York Pantheon.

Sontag, Susan. 1979. *Illness as metaphor.* New York: Vintage.

Spiro, Howard M. 1998. *The power of hope: A doctor's perspective*, New Haven, CT: Yale University Press.

Trabant, Jürgen, ed. 2005. *Sprache der Geschichte.* München: Oldenbourg.

Vigarello, Georges. 1988. *Concepts of cleanliness: Changing attitudes in France since the Middle Ages.* Cambridge: Cambridge University Press.

3 Medicine as practice and culture

The analysis of border regimes and the necessity of a hermeneutics of physical bodies

Gesa Lindemann

In order to understand the relevance of a social science approach to bio-medicine, I will proceed in three steps. First, I will give a short outline of what I understand to be the crucial features of a social science perspective, and I will show how a social science perspective and the interdisciplinary approach of science and technology studies (STS) can be involved in a fruitful discussion beyond the established lines of the Bloor–Latour debates. It is one of the main questions within these debates whether, next to human beings, other entities can be social actors, too.[1] I will argue that sociological theory is implicitly less focused on human actors than Bloor suggested. Furthermore, I suggest that an analysis of how the actor status is distributed can profit from a sociological perspective. Second, I will describe why the analysis of biomedicine is important to scholars in the social sciences by introducing the concept of "biomedical border regimes."

Since biomedicine is not only a culture but also a physical practice, I will finally introduce the methodology of a hermeneutics of physical bodies. The relevance of my theoretical and methodological considerations will be described with reference to the empirical analysis of the treatment of patients in intensive care units.

THE BASIC ASSUMPTION OF A SOCIAL SCIENCE PERSPECTIVE: A FORMAL THEORY OF THE SOCIAL

Despite the heterogeneity of the theories and methods in the social sciences, the different approaches converge at one point. They all presuppose that their subject—social phenomena—can be characterized by certain general features. Contemporary sociological theories refer to a dyadic constellation as the systematic starting point of their conceptualization of the social. The complex relationship between at least two entities is understood as the basis of the development of a novel order that functions as a mediating structure between the involved parties. The decisive property of this order is such that it cannot be reduced to the actions of a single entity. Georg Simmel (1908/1983) was the first to formulate this assumption: He understood the "interaction" (Wechselwirkung) within the relationship between an I and a You as a necessary precondition for the emergence of qualitatively new phenomena, the sociating process with its structuring social forms. Max Weber (1921–1922/1980) viewed social formations in a similar way; he considered the legitimate order, for example, as something that enables the actor to act within social relationships. Comparable patterns of thought can be found in the works of George H. Mead. He understood symbols and the "generalized other" as mediating structures within the relationship between Ego and Alter (Mead 1934/1967). A key concept of Talcott Parson's theory is that of "double contingency" between two actors Ego and Alter (Parsons 1968).[2]

The consensual dyadic concept of the social in these works and in social science theory in general can be characterized as two interacting entities— Ego and Alter. The concept assumes that in the interactional situation, Ego perceives Alter and develops expectations concerning Alter's behavior in the course of the interaction. If Alter correspondingly perceives Ego and develops expectations regarding Ego's behavior, then both are according their behavior with one another's. Ego and Alter find themselves in a situation of simple contingency, since the behavior of the experienced other is uncertain and contingent. But things are even more complex.

Ego observes Alter as a Self that distinguishes itself from its environment and aligns its actions with its perceptions. Furthermore, Ego experiences itself as a Self that exists as a perceiving and acting Self in the environment of Alter. As such, Ego is a Self which is observed by Alter as a Self that observes Alter. In this way, Ego and Alter are each a Self that (1) perceives its environment; (2) perceives the existence of another Self in its environment; and (3) experiences that it is perceived by its counterpart as a Self that experiences its counterpart as a perceiving Self. In such a highly complex relationship, Ego and Alter experience each other mutually as real others; this phenomenon is constitutive for sociological analysis.

Since Ego and Alter are subjects, their behaviors become mutually conditional upon each other in a complex way. Ego and Alter must expect from each other that the other's mediation of perceiving and acting is dependent upon the way in which their respective counterpart presents itself. From the perspective of Ego, this means that Ego in its own behavior incorporates the behavior of Alter by expecting that Alter expects Ego to make its own behavior dependent upon Alter. A double uncertainty emerges. Since Ego and Alter are both subjects trying to adjust their actions according to their mutual expectation-expectations, that is, to the expected expectations of the other, they cannot know for sure how the other will behave. Furthermore, they even cannot know how to behave themselves, since their behavior is dependent on the other. This double uncertainty exists for both Ego and Alter.

In social theory, entities which are involved in such a highly complex relationship are considered as social actors or social persons in a sociological sense. Within the framework of a relationship characterized by expectation-expectations, social persons produce symbols and social meanings, and their relationship to each other is structured by a symbolic order.

Social persons are engaged in a process of mutual interpretation and reinterpretation, that is, Ego interprets Alter and Alter interprets Ego's interpretation of Alter, and so on. In this process is developed what has to be considered as a valid interpretation for both participants. An interpretation consists of two steps which must be distinguished. First, Ego has to decide whether an encountered body has to be treated as a counterpart bearing expectations or not. This decision is important since it defines the relationship between Ego and Alter. Once the counterpart is considered as someone with expectations, Ego begins to determine Alter's situational expectations through a second interpretation, that is, deciding which expectations apply for Alter's perception of Ego and vice versa. However, Ego cannot directly observe the intentions and expectations of Alter, nor can it directly observe Alter's perceptions of Ego. Alter is only indirectly accessible to the perceiving Ego. For this reason, Ego depends on interpreting the way in which Alter appears as an indication of how Alter relates to its environment. In order to know something about Alter, Ego must interpret the latter's gestures and speech. This is the known part of the interpretive process which—in contrast to the first step of interpretation—has been widely observed and theorized in social theory.

Whereas in STS it is questioned whether only human beings can be social actors, it is taken for granted in sociological theory that only conscious human beings are social actors or social persons. Focusing on the first step of interpretation offers the opportunity to involve STS and sociological theory in a discussion—beneficial for both sides. Instead of following the established lines of the debates between the more traditional sociological approach of the sociology of scientific knowledge (SSK) on the one side and the actor-network theory (ANT) on the other side, I suggest that sociological theory can learn how contingent the construction of the actor status is, and STS can profit from the precision of theory construction offered by social theory.

An advantage offered by sociological theory is the insight that the status of being an actor has a paradoxical structure. The first step of interpretation is a foundational interpretation which establishes a border; by this interpretation, the realm of social persons is delimited concretely. But to read the act of classifying an entity as a person as an interpretation inevitably leads to an inextricable paradox: Insofar as the entity is interpreted as a person, the fact of being a person depends upon the interpretative act of Ego. But Ego can only relate to Alter as a person if Alter is an autonomous being, that is, is independent of Ego. To exist in a relationship characterized by expectation-expectations, both Ego and Alter have to experience their counterpart as persons in their own right. But they only exist as persons if they interpret one another as persons. In short: Being a person is dependent on the act of an interpretative ascription, but it cannot be grasped only with reference to the act of an interpretative ascription of the status of a person, since a person has to be a person in his or her own right. This paradoxical structure becomes obvious if one focuses on the relationship of mutual expectation-expectations. This offers a fresh perspective on the problem of being a social person. The empirical analysis of STS scholars has shown that the status of being an actor is ascribed not only to human beings but also to artifacts (Callon & Latour 1992; Latour & Woolgar 1979). The theoretical analysis of the actor status suggests that interpretive ascription is not enough, since ascription cannot account for the actor as an autonomous being; that is, an actor independent of an interpretative ascription. Now the question arises whether that can be corroborated by empirical data.[3]

To date, it is common sense in STS that theories have to be derived from ethnographical data. What I propose here is a methodological shift. I start with a theoretical assumption in the sense of a sensitizing concept (Blumer 1954/1986). The theory serves as a tool which guides the process of collecting and interpreting data. Such a sensitizing concept cannot be falsified or verified, but it can enable interesting observations and descriptions or not. A theoretical construction that takes into account the first step of interpretation draws the attention (1) on the occurrence of border phenomena in social reality, and (2) on the problem that the acknowledgment of the other as a social person has a paradoxical structure as outlined above. I will describe the processes by which social persons and other beings are distinguished as the border regime of a concrete society (Lindemann 2002a).

THE BIOMEDICAL BORDER REGIME

From a social science perspective, biomedicine is a relevant field of research because it is crucial for an analysis of the process of interpretation and reinterpretation. On the one hand, biomedicine plays a crucial role within the border regime of modern societies (the logical first step of interpretation), and on the other hand, biomedical concepts are relevant for how a Self experiences itself and how it comprehends its relations to other selves (the logical second step of interpretation). Since the second point is treated as relevant by many others, I will focus my essay on the first topic: The analysis of biomedicine is crucial for an understanding of modern societies' border regime. This becomes clear if one takes into account that the difference between social persons and other beings is in principle not identical to the difference between living humans and nonhumans. It is a well-stated fact in ethnographical and historical research that in other societies, not only living human beings are treated as social actors, who are engaged in a process of interpretation and reinterpretation. I will give a historical example: Between the end of the thirteenth and the beginning of the eighteenth centuries, animals were treated in European criminal law as responsible actors. They were sued in official trials, which did not differ from trials against humans (Berkenhoff 1937, Evans 1906). Some official documents even stated that the sued animal had confessed its deed. A judge accepted, for example, the confession of a dog, that "he" (the dog) had murdered a child. Thus, a well-educated adult man experienced himself as being interpreted by the sued animal as a mindful actor with intentions and expectations. Otherwise, the judge could not have interpreted a gesture or any other sign from the animal as a confession of the truth.

It was not earlier than the eighteenth century that the circle of social persons was equated—at least in Europe—with the circle of living humans (Lindemann 2001a). Now a new border regime emerged, which must be described as a biomedical border regime (Lindemann 2002a, 2002b, 2003). If only living humans can be social persons in a general valid way, some crucial questions emerge: When does the life of a human begin? When does it end? When is a human alive enough in order to be a social person? And when is a human being dead enough? It is easy to recognize the pressing anthropological border questions, which are forced on us by modern biomedicine. The societal institutions which are concerned with these questions are the state, politics, and law on the one hand and biomedicine on the other hand. In the second half of the nineteenth century, an alliance between state and biomedicine emerged (Lindemann 2003). The state guaranteed that only medical doctors are allowed to establish the fact that a human is dead. Therefore, the end as well as the onset of life became purely biological phenomena.

Taking this into account, it becomes obvious that the modern border regime functions indirectly. It is not the difference between persons and nonpersons which turns out to be the decisive problem; instead, it is the difference between life and the "prealive" and respectively the "postalive" states of a human body. Since biomedical practices contribute to controlling the borders of modern society in that sense, biomedicine becomes one of the most relevant fields for research in the social sciences.

THE FORMAL THEORY AS A CONCEPTUAL TOOL OF EMPIRICAL RESEARCH

In order to outline the methodological problems of such an analysis of modern society's border regime, I will refer to my own research on the borders at the end of life. My study compared the developments of the brain death concept in different scientific cultures in the United States and in Germany (Lindemann 2003), and was concerned with the practice of brain death diagnosis in two intensive care units in Germany (Lindemann 2001b, 2002b).[4] The latter includes an analysis of the interactions between medical staff and patients. Such an analysis raises difficult methodological problems.

In a mediated manner, intensive care patients are social persons. They are treated, because it is expected that they expect the doctor to treat them according to the standards of medicine. As long as the human body is interpreted by medical professionals as being alive, it is included in the practices of communication. A living human body communicates a message, which can be translated into words: "Help me! I allow you to use invasive measures to help me": It is observable, at least in Germany, that within the framework of the communicative processes a human body cannot not communicate this message. Obviously, the precondition of such a communication is the interpretation of the patient's body as a body being alive. The task of giving a description of this interpretation requires a different methodology, since such an analysis is not concerned with communication but with the practical medical diagnosis and treatment of physical bodies. This is especially true for an analysis of medical treatment of patients in intensive care units.

I will start with a brief description of the state of intensive care patients. They lie in bed, and they do not speak or communicate in any other way. In addition, they hardly move, either because they have been anesthetized or because they are comatose. They are usually put on a respirator, and their bodies are connected to several measuring devices and some automatic syringes, which continually pump drugs into the bloodstream. In order to analyze the physical interaction with a patient's body, a hermeneutics of physical bodies is required. If such a hermeneutics is not adopted, a patient becomes invisible to sociologists. Strauss et al. describe a patient as inert if he or she is comatose or temporarily nonsentient (Strauss et al. 1985: 9). According to Strauss, the inert patient cannot participate in health work. Thus, he or she becomes invisible as an acting being. Zussman has put it laconically: "In intensive care the patient vanishes" (Zussman 1992: 43). The question I wish to pose is this: How would a hermeneutics of physical bodies have to work in order to make the patient visible again? How can social scientists grasp the medical interpretations of the physical body and its activities by which the medical staff establishes that a body is dead, alive, or aware of its environment?

The hermeneutics of physical things is derived from the sensitizing concept, that is, the above mentioned theory of the social and its inherent paradoxical structure of the social person. This theory implies in a very elaborated manner a hermeneutics of physical things. Living human beings are interpreted as social persons with reference to different kinds of physical expressions. These can be observed, and can be taken as an indication of something which is not directly accessible: Intentions and expectations are only accessible insofar as they are expressively realized in, for example, vocal gestures or written language which have to be interpreted as an indication of an entity expressing its intentions and expectations. Thus, there is a paradoxical structure which implies, on the one hand, the interpretation and the interpretive ascription of being a person and, on the other hand, the *Sachverhalt* that a being exists autonomously as a person whose expressive realization has to be interpreted. Communication would be impossible without assuming this paradoxical structure. A similar structure can be found within the medical treatment of a patient. The medical staff has a positive knowledge of the physical appearance of the patient, that is, of the visible, palpable, and in many ways divisible gestalt (in the sense of classic gestalt theory). In order to know whether the patient is alive, a doctor has to interpret the gestalt, that is, he or she takes the physical appearance as an indication of something that is not directly accessible. This is true not only for the interpretation of the gestalt as a person, but also for the reading of the gestalt as a living being. To emphasize the similarity of these interpretations, I would like to introduce the term *ou-topian counterpart*. Ou-topian is to be understood literally in the sense of an ou topos: a nowhere place. Something ou-topian has no place within the topology of positive knowledge. Perceived beings are an ou-topian counterpart insofar as they have no determined place within the realm of positive knowledge.

THE PATIENT AS AN OU-TOPIAN
EXPRESSIVE COUNTERPART

Since medical textbooks do not provide a definition of either life or awareness, a physician has to work on terra incognita. The lacking definition of life becomes obvious when looking at a German textbook on physiology:

> Even a virus has a kind of life. An amoeba, a tree, a dog, a person: all of them are alive. The science of physiology attempts to shed light on the physical and chemical factors responsible for the onset, development and sustaining of life. Thereby, the question of what is actually happening serves merely as the starting-off point for the question of how it happens. Thus the physiologist asks: How do ions manage to pass through cell membranes, and what are the signals by means of which cells communicate with each another? How does one fish survive in fresh water, and another in salt water?... How do our kidneys function, our muscles, our eyes, indeed even...our brain? (Klinke & Silbernagl 1996: 2)[5]

We learn that it is the quality of being alive that distinguishes animate beings from inanimate ones. Yet we are not told anywhere in the book about what life is. Other textbooks do not even mention life explicitly, but simply regard it as an unquestioned precondition for medicoscientific and therapeutic activities. Although none of the medical staff really knows what life is, everyone knows how the gestalt of a body must physically appear in order to be interpreted as a living being or as a body aware of itself and its environment. Being alive is considered as the necessary precondition for any medical intervention. However, since life is not really explicated, the living being falls not within but outside the topology of medical knowledge. The patient as a living being is thus an ou-topian counterpart and is, as such, the very precondition for any medical intervention.

These preliminary remarks highlight the value of the following interpretative model for sociological theory. I would like to explain this model by presenting further data from my ethnographical research in two intensive care units. The model differentiates among three levels: (1) the patient as an ou-topian counterpart; (2) the patient as a perceptible gestalt; and (3) discrete elements, that is, results of clinical and laboratory tests. The starting point for any medical intervention, from diagnosis to treatment, is always the gestalt. There are two levels of meaning to the relationship between the gestalt of the patient and the patient as an ou-topian counterpart: The physician takes the gestalt as an indication of the fact that the patient is alive, and the physician experiences the gestalt as an expressive realization of the patient as a living being. In an intensive care unit, it is sometimes difficult to know whether a patient is alive or not. Under such circumstances, the reading of the gestalt is not an ad hoc interpretation (like in classical gestalt theory), but a time-consuming diagnosis. The patient is subjected to various clinical and laboratory tests. Clinical tests such as the tests of reflexes or auscultation are performed within the scope of the physical interaction between the doctor and the patient. In order to carry out a lab test, the gestalt has to be divided into parts which have to be compatible with the laboratory. The parts then leave the intensive care unit and return as results. The results of the various tests form discrete elements. As such, they are scientifically and therapeutically insignificant. In order to make them meaningful, they have to be arranged into a plausible gestalt. The integration of every single discrete element into a specific diagnosis aims to establish a certain disease as the cause for the body that is in a certain state. However, this ideal goal is only rarely achieved in everyday practice. A gestalt that succeeds in integrating most of the discrete elements is seen as a good diagnosis.

As isolated parts and test results, the patient is sometimes scattered all over the hospital; the body reacting to reflexes stays in the ward, the computerized tomography scans are provided in the radiology department, the blood stays in the hematological laboratory, and so on. All these scattered discrete elements have to be assigned to the patient—as an ou-topian counterpart. Once they are identified as signs of the patient X, the discrete elements are ready to be arranged into the gestalt.[6] Each additional test can cause the problem of making it impossible to integrate the discrete elements into a plausible gestalt; thus, using too many tests can question diagnostic certainty. In brain death diagnosis, for example, I experienced the following situation: Everything seemed to be clear. The patient did not react by reflexes to the prescribed stimuli. She did not even react to the most severe pain stimuli, such as pricking with the needle of a syringe through the septum. Suddenly, a problem occurred. The diagnosis of brain death regularly includes an analysis of the blood in order to determine the level of carbonic acid. Although it is not an essential part of brain death diagnosis, the level of blood sugar is determined routinely by members of the medical staff in the observed intensive care unit. In the described situation, this test was not really indispensable. Nevertheless, the staff decided to apply it. Once applied, the results of the test had to be taken into consideration. In that case, the results indicated a diabetic coma. This meant that one could not exclude any longer that the nonreaction to the stimuli of brain death diagnosis was due to the very high level of blood sugar. In terms of diagnostic certainty, the test was irritating. The patient was too ill to remain with the diagnosis of death. After treating the high level of blood sugar, the procedures of brain death diagnosis were performed once more. Based on the results of these procedures, it became possible to establish the diagnosis of brain death. Afterwards, several organs were taken from the patient's body.

After finishing every prescribed test of brain death diagnosis, the results have to be assigned to the patient, and are then arranged into a plausible gestalt. For example, a patient suffering from intracerebral bleeding (which causes an incurable pressure within the skull and thereby a deadly damage of the brain and the brain stem) and a patient suffering from a too high level of blood sugar can appear very similar. Nevertheless, the two diseases would be a different diagnostic gestalt, since such a gestalt has a time structure. It necessarily includes a past which caused the actual physical state. The past of a patient in a diabetic coma is very different from the past of a patient suffering from intracranial bleeding. A similar actual appearance does not guarantee the similarity of the diagnostic gestalt.

Performing the tests and arranging them into a plausible gestalt are activities exerted by the medical staff. The result of their activity, the arranged gestalt, will be interpreted by asking if it indicates the presence of the patient as a living being or not. If the physical appearance is interpreted as being alive, the arranged gestalt—the result of the physicians' actions—is seen as an expressive realization of the patient's life, that is, the result of the patient's own activity. If the physical appearance is interpreted as an indication of the patient's death, the arranged gestalt is seen as an indication of the nonexistence of the patient as a being whose life is expressively realized within the gestalt. The equivocal relationship between the gestalt and the patient as an ou-topian counterpart becomes an unequivocal one: The gestalt indicates the presence of the patient, who is not a living being but an inanimate body.

The tests and their arrangement into a conclusive gestalt belong to the realm of the positive knowledge, which is mastered by the medical staff. To read the gestalt as an indication of being inanimate/dead, alive, or aware—or as a person—implies a qualitative leap to what lies outside the topology of mastered positive knowledge. The medical practice of interpreting physical bodies cannot avoid its counterparts as ou-topian beings. The expressive realization of life refers to the patient as an ou-topian counterpart who expresses him or herself autonomously in the physical gestalt. Thus, the diagnosis of the patient as being alive has a paradoxical structure. On the one hand, it is the result of the interpretative ascription of medical doctors, but on the other hand, the gestalt is understood as the autonomous expressive realization of the patient as a living being.

CONCLUSION

The ethnography, the data of which I have presented here, was theory driven. The collection of data and its interpretation were guided by a concept which was derived from sociological theory. To take into account the first step of interpretation served as a concept which made the analysis sensitive for (1) border phenomena in social reality, and (2) the paradoxical structure of the acknowledgment of the other as a social person. In both respects, the theoretical concept has worked efficiently. The diagnosis of death could be identified as a border regime, which delimits the realm of social persons.

In the case of the analysis of border regimes, the analysis transcends the limitations of traditional sociological analysis. Sociological analysis of the treatment of intensive care patients—as it is effected, for example, by Strauss and Zussman—is usually restricted to interactions structured by mutual expectation-expectations. Such studies only address the second step of interpretation but do not look at the elementary first step by which it is decided which entities have to be treated as social persons. Focusing on the logical first step of interpretation broadens the scope of the sociological analysis in a systematic way. The patient as a living being is made visible. An unconscious patient is an actor whose expressivity contributes to accomplishing the crucial features of the situation. If the patient's expressivity would stop, the features of the situation would dramatically change. A dead patient would at once be removed from the ward—either he or she would be brought to the morgue or prepared for harvesting organs. Furthermore, the elementary physical expressivity of being alive shows that it has a paradoxical structure similar to the acknowledgment of being an actually communicating alter Ego.

One intention of this essay was to involve science studies, especially ANT, and sociological theory into a discussion. The advantage for sociological theory should have become clear: to extend the circle of actors beyond the circle of self-conscious human beings. With reference to ANT, the advantage of my approach lies in making the concept of being an actor more differentiated. Up to now, usually two different actor positions are differentiated: human persons and artifacts. To focus systematically on the first step of interpretation reveals that a more differentiated concept is required: Besides the actor positions of human social persons on the one hand, and artifacts on the other hand, the actor position of the body being alive should be included not only in the analysis of actor networks[7] but also in any social analysis of technoscientific and biomedical practices.

NOTES

1. The problem of the actor lies at the core of the debates between the strong program (Bloor 1991, 1999a, 1999b; Collins & Yearley 1992) and the actor-network theory (Latour 1991/1995, 1999; Callon & Latour 1992).
2. Although Niklas Luhmann (1984) interpreted the concept of double contingency differently from Parsons, he continued the tradition of using a dyadic key concept in order to understand the emergence of a novel type of order, which he described as autopoietic social systems.
3. See the methodological considerations in Callon and Latour (1992). A more detailed analysis of the Latourian methodology reveals that its basic problem is not that it includes nonhumans as actors. On the contrary, the foundational problem is that the Latourian methodology remains anthropocentric. Humans (technicians and engineers) are the crucial actors who can ascribe the status of an actor to nonhumans, whereas the nonhumans cannot ascribe the status of an actor to a human being in a symmetrical way; see Lindemann (2002b: ch. 2; 2005: 70ff.; 2006).
4. Lock (2002) has offered a detailed comparison of "brain death" in Japan and the United States. It would be an interesting topic to discuss the differences of biomedical cultures in Japan, Germany, and the United States. Nevertheless, I restrict myself in this context to unfolding the relationship of theory and empirical data.
5. Translation by Gesa Lindemann and Allison Brown.
6. This analysis corroborates in some respects the results of Annemarie Mol's (2003) ethnography of atherosclerosis. She argued that different subdisciplines in medicine produce multiple bodies. This is equivalent to what I describe as the dissection of the body necessary to perform the diagnosis. However, concerning the integration of the dissected parts into a diagnostic gestalt, my account is different from Mol's. This is mainly due to the concept of the patient as an ou-topian counterpart, which has no equivalent in her account of the multiple body.
7. Mol (2003) talks about social persons as experiencing bodies. Such bodies can talk and go from one medical department to another. Bodies merely being alive are different: They cannot talk, they cannot move, they are simply alive, and as such they are actors. Elsewhere, I have shown that a fourth actor position can be identified, the body being aware of itself and its environment, which can be clearly differentiated from the body being alive and the actor position of the social person (Lindemann 2002b: ch. 5).

REFERENCES

Berkenhoff, Hans Albert. 1937. *Tierstrafe, Tierbannung und Rechtsrituelle Tiertötung im Mittelalter.* Strasbourg.
Bloor, David. 1991. *Knowledge and social imagery*, 2nd ed. Chicago: University of Chicago Press.
———. 1999a. Anti-Latour. *Studies in History and Philosophy of Science* 30: 81–112.

58   Gesa Lindemann

———. 1999b. Reply to Bruno Latour. *Studies in History and Philosophy of Science* 30:31–36.

Blumer, Herbert. 1954/1986. What is wrong with social theory? In *Symbolic Interactionism: Perspective and method*, edited by Herbert Blumer, 140–52. Berkeley: University of California Press.

Callon, Michel, and Bruno Latour. 1992. Don't throw the baby out with the bath school! A Reply to Collins and Yearley. In *Science as practice and culture*, edited by Andrew Pickering, 343–68. Chicago: University of Chicago Press.

Collins, Harry M., and Steven Yearley. 1992. Epistemological chicken. In *Science as practice and culture*, edited by Andrew Pickering, 301–26. Chicago: University of Chicago Press.

Evans, Edward P. 1906. *The criminal prosecution and capital punishment of animals*. London: Faber and Faber.

Klinke, Rainer, and Stefan Silbernagl. 1996. *Lehrbuch der Physiologie*. 2nd ed. Stuttgart: Thieme.

Latour, Bruno. 1991/1995. *Wir sind nie modern gewesen*. Berlin: Akademie Verlag.

———. 1999. For David Bloor...and beyond: A reply to David Bloor's "Anti-Latour." *Studies in History and Philosophy of Science* 30: 113–29.

Latour, Bruno, and Steve Woolgar. 1979. *Laboratory life: The social construction of scientific facts*. London: Sage.

Lindemann, Gesa. 2001a. Die reflexive Anthropologie des Zivilisationsprozesses. *Soziale Welt* 52, no. 2: 181–98.

———. 2001b. Die Interpretation "hirntot." In *Hirntod. Zur Kulturgeschichte der Todesfeststellung*, edited by Thomas Schlich and Claudia Wiesemann, 318–43. Frankfurt am Main: Suhrkamp.

———. 2002a. Kritik der Soziologie. *Deutsche Zeitschrift für Philosophie* 50, no. 2: 227–45.

———. 2002b. *Die Grenzen des Sozialen. Zur sozio-technischen Konstruktion von Leben und Tod in der Intensivmedizin*. München: Fink.

———. 2003. *Beunruhigende Sicherheiten. Zur Genese des Hirntodkonzepts*. Konstanz: Universitätsverlag.

———. 2005. The analysis of the borders of the social world: A challenge for sociological theory. *Journal for the Theory of Social Behavior* 35:69–98.

———. 2006. Die Emergenzfunktion und die konstitutive Funktion des Dritten. Perspektiven einer kritisch-systematischen Theorieentwicklung. *Zeitschrift für Soziologie* 35:82–101.

Lock, Margaret. 2002. *Twice dead: Organ transplants and the reinvention of death*. Berkeley: University of California Press.

Luhmann, Niklas. 1984. *Soziale Systeme. Grundriß einer allgemeinen Theorie*. Frankfurt am Main: Suhrkamp.

Mead, George H. 1934/1967. *Mind, self, and society*. Chicago: University of Chicago Press.

Mol, Annemarie. 2003. *The body multiple: Ontology in medical practice*. Durham, NC: Duke University Press.

Parsons, Talcott. 1968. Interaction: Social interaction. In *International encyclopedia of the social sciences*, vol. 7, 429–41. New York: Macmillan/Free Press.

Simmel, Georg. 1908/1983. *Soziologie. Untersuchungen über die Formen der Vergesellschaftung*. Berlin: Duncker und Humblot.

Strauss, Anselm, Shizuko Fagerhaugh, Barbara Suczek, and Carolyn Wiener. 1985. *Social organization of medical work*. Chicago: University of Chicago Press.

Weber, Max. 1921–1922/1980. *Wirtschaft und Gesellschaft*. Tübingen: Mohr.

Zussman, Robert. 1992. *Intense care: Medical ethics and the medical profession*. Chicago: University of Chicago Press.

Part II
Epistemic practices and material culture(s)

4 The future is now
Locating biomarkers for dementia

Margaret Lock

The molecular vision of life that predominated during the second half of the twentieth century, culminating recently in the mapping of the human genome, is grounded in a mechanistic biology, one primary objective of which is to enable the engineering of bodies and minds (Kay 1993: 17). This particular form of molecularization is deterministic, one assumption being that knowledge about specific genes makes possible reliable predictions about the occurrence of disease. As part of this endeavor, technological innovations since the mid-1980s have facilitated the genetic testing and screening of individuals, with both negative and positive consequences (Duster 1990; Kitcher 1996). However, this particular form of molecular biology, although its approach remains valid for single-gene disorders, shows many signs of being on the wane. Theorizing and research into susceptibility genes[1] implicated in complex diseases and behaviors have brought about a fundamental transformation in molecular biology, on the order of a paradigm shift, with enormous potential consequences for clinical care of all kinds, including the genetic testing of individuals.

When mapping the human genome, involved scientists set aside approximately 98 percent of the DNA they had isolated, labeling it as "junk" because it did not conform with their idea of how the blueprint for life was assumed to work. Since the announcement in early 2001 that the Human Genome Project was more or less complete, things have changed dramatically and junk DNA, thrust summarily to one side in order to focus on the task of mapping only those genes that code directly for proteins, can no longer be ignored. It was recently noted in *Scientific American*, for example, that

> new evidence...contradicts conventional notions that genes...are the sole mainspring of hereditary and the complete blueprint for all life. Much as dark matter influences the fate of galaxies, dark parts of the genome exert control over the development and the distinctive traits of all organisms, from bacteria to humans....[S]ome scientists now suspect that much of what makes one person, and one species, different

from the next are variations in the gems hidden within our "junk" DNA. (Gibbs 2003: 48)

This junk is composed largely of RNA that does not code for protein production but, even so, is deeply implicated in gene expression and regulation, and so must now be sifted through (Eddy 2001; Mattick 2003, 2004). The result is that we have entered an era, almost overnight, in which the "dark" parts of the genome are starting to fluoresce.

The activities of noncoding RNA (ncRNA) are believed to comprise the most comprehensive regulatory system in complex organisms; ncRNA functions to create the "architecture" of organisms, without which chaos would reign (Mattick 2003). To this end, ncRNA has been shown to profoundly affect the timing of processes that take place during development, including stem cell maintenance, cell proliferation, apoptosis (programmed cell death), and the onset of cancer and other complex ailments (Petronis 2001). Consequently, the research interests of molecular biology are no longer confined largely to mapping structure, but have expanded to unraveling the mechanisms of cell and organ function through time. Central to this endeavor is to understand gene regulation—above all how, and under what circumstances, genes are switched "on" and "off."[2] In this rapidly proliferating science known as epigenetics, organized complexity is recognized, and activities of the cell, rather than simply those of genes, are the primary targets of investigation, although the effects of evolutionary, historical, and environmental variables on cellular activity, developmental processes, health, and disease are freely acknowledged.

This emerging knowledge has exploded the central dogma on which molecular genetics was founded. Metaphors associated with the mapping of the human genome—the Book of Life, the Code of Codes, the Holy Grail, and so on—are entirely outmoded. The result is that gene fetishism—never embraced wholeheartedly by all involved scientists (see Berg 1991 and Davis 1990, to name just two)—is now clearly on the wane among many, perhaps the majority of, experts. DNA is not, after all, a blueprint for the organism. The gene has been dethroned as "part physicist's atom and part Plato's soul" (Fox Keller 2000a: 277), and can no longer pass as the fundamental animating force of human life. Ironically, it is the same technologies of molecularization that enabled systematic manipulation of DNA that are now causing the undoing of the genotype/phenotype dogma that drove the reductionistic approach to genetics dominant for the past fifty years. The current "definitional disarray of the gene" (Fox Keller 2000a: 274; see also Rheinberger 1995) was brought to a head by the findings of the Human Genome Project, and "genes have come to remind, at least some biologists, of the organism, pointing to its peculiarly biological as distinct from its strictly biochemical properties"—in other words, "we might say that the 'organism' has been disinterred from its earlier submission inside the material entity" (Fox Keller 2000a: 275).

With the cell at center stage, gene-gene, gene-protein, and gene-environment interactions cannot be ignored, and biological pathways are no longer thought of as necessarily linear or unidirectional. A space has been opened up between genotype and phenotype that was partially recognized one hundred years ago, but conveniently set to one side. Commenting on these developments, the biologist Richard Lewontin has this to say:

> Unlike planets, which are extremely large, or electrons, which are extremely small and internally homogenous, living organisms are intermediate in size and internally heterogenous. They are composed of a number of parts with different properties that are in dynamic interaction with one another and the parts are, in turn, composed of yet smaller parts with their own interactions and properties. Moreover, they change their shapes and properties during their lifetimes, developing from a fertilized egg to a mature adult, ending finally sans teeth, sans hair, sans everything. In short: organisms are a changing nexus of a large number of weakly determining interacting forces. (Lewontin 2003: 39)

Lewontin wonders if biology is inevitably a story of "different strokes for different folks," a collection of exquisitely detailed descriptions of diverse forms and functions down to the molecular level; or, from "this booming, buzzing confusion," can a biologist derive some general claims that are freed from the dirty particulars of each case? Not laws, of course, but perhaps at least some widely shared characteristics? Lewontin agrees with Fox Keller (2002) that history and epistemology both speak against this and that, as far as making sense of life is concerned, all our models, metaphors, and machines, while they have contributed much to our understanding, provide neither unity nor completeness. On the contrary: Facing up to complexity is the order of the day, although many obdurate problems continue to be studiously avoided, and, more disconcerting, much of what was understood as settled with respect to the function of genes must now be revised.

An interview with the CEO of Perlegen Sciences, published in part in *Genetic Engineering News* (Dutton 2003), makes it clear that, on the basis of revelations about complexity, molecular genomics is at an impasse: "the dream is to identify genetic markers for disease by sequencing the genome of hundreds of thousands of people with and without a given disease. As yet, though, this is not practical." This same magazine notes that genomics and proteomics have not thus far resulted in improved diagnostics or therapeutics (see also Angell 2004), and an employee of Curagen (Dutton 2003: 4) is cited as stating,

> Last year was the worst year in a decade in terms of numbers of new drugs approved by the FDA. Only one of these acted specifically against

a newly identified target from the human genome. The pharmaceutical industry is stalled.

Another interviewee added, "[E]ven if I could sequence your own personal genome, there's not much you could do with the raw sequence information today."

GREEDY REDUCTIONISM

A critical review of the history of genetics from the late nineteenth century (Fox Keller 2000b; Sapp 1983) shows how we have for more than one hundred years been on a path of oversimplification. Disciplinary battles of the day were, as always, struggles for power and authority in which the creation of a genotype/phenotype distinction—a perceptual split between structure and its expression—was to win out over earlier ideas about inheritance that were disparagingly called the "transmission conception of heredity," in which it was assumed that personal qualities and behaviors were passed on from generation to generation. Kerr et al. (1998) and Lock, Freeman et al. (2006a) have shown that the "transmission concept of heredity" continues to be made use of by many, perhaps the majority of, people in their everyday lives, but adoption of the genotype/phenotype distinction in the emerging profession of genetics was to eliminate such associative thinking among experts and swing the pendulum very far in the direction of genetic determinism. By the early twentieth century, genetics had been likened by its founder, the Danish scientist Wilhelm Johannsen, to the "hard" science of chemistry (1923). And the hope was later expressed by H. E. Armstrong, writing in the 1930s, that "some day, perhaps, biography will be written almost in terms of structural chemistry, and the doctrine of descent stated in terms of the permutations and combinations affected between genes"; any other order of explanation was regarded as superfluous (Armstrong 1931: 238).

Daniel Dennet argues that scientists exhibit "greedy reductionism" when "in their zeal to explain too much too fast, [they] under-estimate complexity, trying to skip whole layers or levels of theory in their rush to fasten everything securely to the foundation" (1995: 82). The seeds were sown for this type of reductionism once the genotype/phenotype distinction became dogma, a position that was then built upon later in the famous 1953 publication of Watson and Crick, "The Structure of DNA," which formed the groundwork for the Central Dogma of the new molecular biology.

As is well-known, Watson and Crick argued for a unidirectional flow of information from DNA to RNA to protein to phenotype, thus consolidating the power of the gene. Profoundly influenced from the 1950s by computer technology and the dazzle of the information sciences, the idea of the genome as an informational template was advanced by reifying the gene itself and trivializing everything else. Any possible contribution to the phenotype made by the environment internal to the organism, most significantly that of individual cells, and the response of the organism as a whole to changing environments was dismissed as so much flotsam (Fox Keller 2002).

Gabriel Gudding notes that the disappearance of the body in molecular genetics over the past decade is associated with new technologies that enable rapid DNA analysis and permit a massive redeployment of agency and morality to the gene (1996). He reminds us how, increasingly, DNA evidence is used as the irrefutable mark of identity, whether in the courtroom as forensic evidence, or in determining if a female athlete is really what she claims to be. Our biographies are in part, at least, written in terms of structural chemistry, and the quest to sequence thousands of genomes—human, animal, and plant—is rapidly being accomplished, although frequently the emerging findings were not as predicted, creating surprises in terms of both the length of genomes and the extensive DNA correspondences among them.

Despite the hype associated with the sequencing of the human genome, with its misplaced metaphors of mapping and the unveiling of the Secret of Life, even before sequencing had commenced, the majority of involved experts knew that mapping was only a small part of the story, and when the human genome was first more or less completed, knowledgeable commentators stated that the resultant map was like being handed the equivalent of a list of parts for a Boeing 747, but with no idea as to how they go together and no awareness of the principles of aeronautics; the map represents a reduction of life to structure alone, and permits no insight into function.

SCALING DOWN COMPLEXITY

In practice, for the majority of basic science researchers, elucidation of the complexity associated with function consists in an effort to clarify what takes place in the hypothetical "space" between genotype and phenotype. The majority of researchers working in molecular genetics today acknowledge that the environment and social variables play crucial roles in modifying organisms; even so, these variables are black-boxed in preference for an approach that remains resolutely concerned with interactions internal to the material body. Most modeling continues, therefore, to be reductionistic and deliberately oversimplified, but characterization of this research as one of genetic determinism is no longer apt.

In psychiatry, for example, Irving Gottesman suggests that models of complex genetic disorders "predict a ballet choreographed interactively over time [among] genotype, environment, and epigenetic factors which give rise to a particular phenotype" (1994: S27). In the early 1970s, Gottesman and Shields, in their investigations of schizophrenia, inspired by publications in insect biology, created a concept of "endophenotypes" that they described as "internal phenotypes" discoverable by a "biochemical test or microscopic examination." Their claim is that endophenotypes provide the means for identifying the "downstream" traits or facets of clinical phenotypes, as well as the "upstream" consequences of gene effects (Gottesman & Shields 1972). Little was made of this concept until recently, but references to it in psychiatric genetics are now common, and it is also beginning to appear in publications in the neurosciences and other human science disciplines. Gottesman (1994: S32) concedes that similar terms in current use—"intermediate phenotype," "biological marker" or "biomarker," "subclinical trait," and "vulnerability marker" —are essentially synonymous with the endophenotype concept, but he wants to limit use of this latter term to those cases where specific heritability indicators are fulfilled. In contrast, biomarkers, he argues, may be the products of environmental, epigenetic, or multifactorial effects.

This shift in emphasis constitutes an epistemological move away from determinism, and with it hopes have been raised for refining diagnostic categories—for being able to classify, for example, schizophrenia, bipolar disorder, and so on into clearly differentiated subtypes and to produce tailor-made pharmacogenetic medications for these subtypes. But, as noted above, so far there have been virtually no deliverables.

In the following section, I turn to the condition of dementia, in particular to Alzheimer's disease (AD), as an illustrative example of how the epigenetic approach to complex disease is being played out in basic science research and the clinic. Routinization of genotyping and tracking of biomarkers are now customary in memory clinics where dementia patients are managed, but to date patients and their families are not informed about the results, and blood collection and other tests are carried out under research protocols in which informed consent forms specify that biological samples are donated for research purposes only, and not as part of clinical care. In the concluding section, I will discuss findings from interviews with volunteers in a randomized controlled trial in which first-degree relatives of individuals diagnosed with Alzheimer's disease are genotyped and then informed of their results. This National Institutes of Health (NIH) trial was designed with the express purpose of eventually extending such testing to the public at large. Open-ended interviews with volunteers in the trial permit a preliminary glimpse at the social effects of testing for susceptibility genes, notably on the arguments put forward by several social scientists about the long-term impact on subjectivity and identity of being labeled as "genetically at risk" (Novas & Rose 2000).

IN SEARCH OF PRODROMAL DEMENTIA

Media coverage of the death of Ronald Reagan in June 2004 included a newspaper article with the headline "Was That Trademark Smile the First

Sign of Alzheimer's?" The author, a physician, suggested that it is quite possible that Mr. Reagan's entire life history and long-established emotional patterns may have "prepared the ground" for the illness that eventually robbed him of thought, speech, and movement. He stated, "Evidence strongly suggests that a lack of full emotional capacity is a risk factor for the later development of Alzheimer's," and he reminds readers that Reagan had an "alcoholic, unreliable father and an emotionally absent mother" (Maté 2004). This information was linked in the same article with findings from the widely cited Nun's Study, in which participated 678 Catholic sisters who belong to an order called the School Sisters of Notre Dame located in seven regions of the United States. Statements written by these nuns when they were young women about why they wanted to enter the order, carefully stored for decades, were matched with neuropsychiatric assessments administered throughout the latter part of their lives from age seventy-five on, and then subsequently linked to autopsy findings after death (every nun had agreed when she entered the project to donate her brain for autopsy). It is argued on the basis of this study that those individuals who exhibited imagination and complexity in their thinking while young (that is, exhibited "high idea density," in the language of the researchers) were less likely to succumb to Alzheimer's disease when they grew older (Snowdon 2001). This finding was not related to number of years of formal education, and was borne out as the autopsy results gradually accumulated: Ninety percent of those nuns whose brains exhibited extensive damage had shown "low idea density" as twenty year olds. This research gave an enormous boost to what has come to be known as the "cerebral reserve" hypothesis—such reserve being laid down commencing from the time in utero, and drawn on heavily today when theorizing about who is at risk for AD.

Of even greater interest was the finding that a small proportion of the nuns who coped very ably with the neuropsychological battery of tests administered to them turned out at autopsy to have extensive signs of the plaques and tangles assumed, since the time of Alois Alzheimer, to be the pathological hallmarks of the disease. Recent research, including a project in which the brains of deceased centenarians have been autopsied, has yielded similar counterintuitive results (Silver et al. 2001). Conversely, it is also well recognized that a few individuals whose autopsied brains show a relatively small number of anatomical changes exhibit all the behavioral signs of dementia while alive (Swartz et al. 1999).

Adding to the confusion, it is now evident that dementias, perhaps without exception, come in "mixed forms," so that cerebro-vascular dementia is frequently present together with late-onset AD; alternatively, late-onset AD may be mixed with fronto-temporal dementia that causes hallucinations. Yet other permutations and combinations exist among the "dementing disorders," a taxonomic group that includes Creutzfeldt-Jakob disease. Virtually no one today would argue that dementia is a myth, an exemplar of social construction, as was argued by some experts in the not too distant past (Stafford 1991); nor are plaques and tangles fantasy. (Late-onset AD is, however, perhaps a convenient fiction; among medical professionals, it is implicitly recognized as a shifting, unstable target that experts agree must be noted on diagnostic charts as "probable Alzheimer's disease" until such time as an autopsy, if and when it is done, confirms the diagnosis; although, as noted above, even autopsies do not necessarily constitute hard evidence.) After years of attempting to improve both the sensitivity and the specificity of AD diagnoses, even in academic medical centers their accuracy varies between 63 and 90 percent. Meanwhile, at least one clinician/researcher has written an article entitled "The End of Alzheimer's Disease," in which he speculates that in the postgenomic era we will do away with this troublesome label entirely (Whitehouse 2001)—a possibility that is actively opposed, for obvious reasons, by the International Alzheimer Society and its various chapters.

These paradoxes immediately raise the question of the ontological status of late-onset Alzheimer's disease—what is "it," and where exactly does "it" reside? Do the behavioral changes diagnosed on the basis of psychological testing, or the anatomical pathology demonstrated at autopsy, constitute the disease? And how exactly are genes implicated? Many involved scientists and clinicians are sensitive to this taxonomic conundrum, although few, of course, are explicitly concerned with ontology.

PINNING DOWN AD

The UN Population Division estimates that the number of people in the world aged sixty years and older exceeded 635 million in 2002. By mid-century, they will be about 2 billion, assuming starvation and infectious disease do not take an even greater toll than is currently the case. This means that 1 in 3 of us, or even 1 in 2 if the AIDS crisis continues unabated, will be over sixty, and the oldest old are the fastest growing group among the aged. Governments are running scared, and drug companies are hungry for breakthroughs in what is described as the new "pandemic of aging." Fear of being overrun by the demented elderly means that money is available for research; at the same time, genomic technologies have become incrementally more efficient, and knowledge about the molecular mechanisms of AD has advanced. Even so, at present, there are neither sound preventive measures nor any treatments that do more than improve the situation for a few months in some patients—and these effects may well be entirely due to the placebo effect; in other words, caregivers note slight improvements because they are predisposed to do so when they are in charge of handing out medication (Grady 2004).

One result of the present impasse is that dementia research has burgeoned in a new direction. The time span that now interests many researchers extends backwards by two or three decades from the usual age of onset of dementia, and the focus of attention is on people in middle age or even younger; those individuals who, it is believed, may well be beginning to harbor one or more of the endophenotypes currently recognized as candidate biomarkers for the first signs of a preclinical, prodromal stage of dementia (Breitner 1999; DeKosky & Marek 2003).

These elusive biomarkers are now thought of by many as the core, or essence, of the disease. Some scientists, notably epidemiologists interested in the social determinants of health, argue that the presence of such biomarkers may in part be the products of the effects of a combination of a genetic predisposition with specific types of parental behaviors during very early development in utero and infancy that in concert affect the wiring of the infant brain, and hence aptitude for formal education, which in turn further negatively affects the buildup of "cerebral reserve." No one doubts that ultimately age is the greatest risk factor for late-onset AD. These currently fashionable theses are, in effect, finite regressions on age-dependent, individualized, life-course thinking about dementia causality.

A recent article in *Public Health* gives a strong hint that linear modeling such as the above does not tell the whole story. Colin Pritchard and colleagues note in this article that, after controlling for increased life expectancy, the number of deaths due to dementia has soared over the past twenty years in Europe, North America, and Australia. Even more striking is that dementia deaths are occurring at younger ages (Pritchard et al. 2004). These changes may well in part be explained by the application of more rigorous diagnostic procedures. But, Pritchard et al. hypothesize, in addition, that environmental pollutants are taking their toll. If this is the case, it would neatly account for why people with lower levels of education, who are almost without exception exposed to more pollutants, appear to be at increased risk for AD—providing a more cogent argument than the usual one about individuals with only a few years of formal education being vulnerable because they have relatively fewer brain synapses and hence plaques and tangles take their toll on their paltry quota of "cerebral reserve."[3]

That people who do not receive advanced education have fewer synapses in their brains than individuals with many years of formal education is decidedly questionable. Further, it is usually conveniently forgotten by researchers who make such arguments, given the nature of contemporary education, that people with many years of schooling are rather well prepared to deal with the neuropsychiatric tests dispensed at memory clinics and, moreover, that they may well be adept at "covering up" the early signs of dementia, blurring estimations of who is at risk.

Well-known researchers in the world of neurosciences point out that there are, at the moment, essentially two strategies for searching for biomarkers for AD (Daffner & Scinto 2000). Alzheimer's is a condition that is, of course, associated above all else with memory loss. Hence, in one approach, the focus of attention is on the limbic regions of the brain, primarily on the entorhinal cortex and the hippocampus—those parts of the brain associated with memory. Imaging technologies are used to detect these changes. The second major strategy is to monitor the by-products in the blood and cerebrospinal fluid of the very earliest signs of the extraordinarily complex pathophysiological processes associated with AD. Involved researchers freely acknowledge the preliminary nature and limitations of these strategies.

In 1998, a consensus statement entitled "Molecular and Biomedical Markers of Alzheimer's Disease" was released by the Ronald and Nancy Reagan Research Institute of the Alzheimer's Association and the National Institute on Aging Working Group (reproduced in Scinto & Daffner, 2000: 329–348). Such biomarkers, it is noted, should have a sensitivity for detecting AD of over 80 percent and, similarly, a specificity of over 80 percent in order that they can be reliably distinguished from biomarkers associated with other types of dementia—given what has already been spelled out above with respect to fluid taxonomies, this is indeed a challenge! The statement also points out that biomarkers of this kind must be reliable, reproducible, noninvasive, simple to perform, and inexpensive. In other words, the ultimate objective is to isolate markers that can be readily detected in the offices of general practitioners, perhaps even of those GPs whose practices are located in developing countries. The term *biomarker*, as it is used in this consensus report, includes genes, endophenotypes, and clinical phenotypes. Among targeted biomarkers are neuropathological changes associated with the commencement of excess amyloid deposition resulting in plaque formation. A second is excess production of the protein tau—the precursor of tangles. Diagnosis of both these changes requires not only neuroimaging but also an examination of cerebro-spinal fluid—a highly invasive procedure. Direct-to-consumer advertising encourages people to test themselves at home for another biomarker with smell test kits designed to detect changes in the olfactory epithelium. Yet other biomarkers are tracked by means of blood tests that detect misfolded proteins and changes in pupillary responses, in how one writes, in one's gait, and so on—all of which are considered significant by researchers.

Detection of these biomarkers is most common when people are enrolled into clinical trials or when they participate in clinical research in connection with the condition "discovered" in 1994 known as mild cognitive impairment (MCI). This syndrome is the clinical form of prodromal dementia. Described as "a transitional state between the cognition of normal aging and mild dementia," it is freely acknowledged among experts that MCI is heterogeneous; and a good number of experts refuse to recognize it as a condition at all. The hope is, on the basis of findings from clinical trials, to create subtypes of patients—those with MCI who convert to AD, and those whose cognitive decline is regarded as "normal" and who do not progress to outright pathology. Findings from neuroimaging, neuropsychiatric testing, detection of early molecular changes, and genotyping create assemblies of knowledge that constitute this new space of divination. Thoroughly molecularized, this space is resolutely wedded to the idea of an age-related linear decline into pathology that can be differentiated from normal aging on the basis of extensive monitoring. This exhaustive hunt for endophenotypes will, it is hoped, result in the establishment of clear boundaries for, and the normalization of, prodromal, incipient dementia.[4]

This model gives very little attention to consideration of the contributions to ill health made by the social and physical environments of the thousands of people diagnosed with mild cognitive impairment; it pays only lip service to gene-environment interactions, and works on the assumption that the brain is somewhat like a muscle, an organ that needs flexing and exercising regularly. Individual behavior is presumed to be a direct response to synaptic activity (LeDoux 2002), and higher levels of articulation—mind, family interactions, societal responses to aging and dementia, and toxic environments—are cast to one side.

THE GENETICS OF ALZHEIMER'S DISEASE

It has been known for over twenty years that rare autosomal dominant genes are inevitably associated with what is known as "early-onset Alzheimer's disease"; this form of AD—the type that was originally observed by Alois Alzheimer—has long been conceptualized as a "genetic disease," although the age of onset for identical twins can vary by as much as a decade (Tilley et al. 1998). In 1991, one particular polymorphism of the APOE (apolipoprotein E) gene present in all mammals, located in humans on chromosome 19, was associated for the first time with increased risk for the common, late-onset form of AD. This finding forced some second thoughts about the received wisdom of the day, namely, that Alzheimer's disease in older people is "sporadic" and does not "run in families." Recently, as a result of findings from molecular biology, the thinking has shifted yet again.

A fairly broad consensus now exists among researchers that at least three complex molecular pathways lead to a final common pathway, the endpoint of which is Alzheimer's disease, and it is along these contributory pathways that the hunt for other involved genes and for biomarkers is taking place. The first pathway is kick-started by the switching on in early midlife of one of the specific genes associated with early-onset AD. These mutations are found in about 170 families worldwide. A second, much more common pathway involves the APOE gene. This gene has three, and possibly four, polymorphic variations that are distributed unequally but universally among the human population, the APOEε2, ε3, and ε4 alleles. It is the APOEε4 allele that is implicated in risk for AD. Shortly after the first claims were made in the early 1990s about an association between this allele and increased risk for AD, disagreement existed. Today all researchers and clinicians concur that the allele is a susceptibility gene for AD, but that, although significant, it is neither necessary nor sufficient to cause the disease. Most of the research in connection with APOE has been carried out with Caucasian populations, and there is good reason to suspect that the ε4 allele can be protective in environments where gene pools other than those constituted by Caucasian DNA are dominant, making for further complexity (Corbo & Scacchi 1999). Clinical research in connection with the ε4 allele shows that when it is implicated in AD, exactly the same "final common pathway" is involved as that set in motion by the autosomal dominant genes, but these changes become manifest later in life (Selkoe 2002).

Given that in at least 50 percent of diagnosed cases of late-onset AD, patients do not have the APOEε4 allele, there must be at least one other pathway to AD. Such a pathway is constituted, it is assumed, by mutually interactive genes and noncoding DNA in conjunction with environmental factors internal or external to the body. This third alternative also results in the same final common pathway, with the typical end result of plaques, tangles, and cell loss. Given that as yet "undiscovered" genes are undoubtedly implicated, gene hunting continues to be important among researchers, and numerous "candidate genes" are being investigated for their possible contribution to AD.

Two geneticists of neurodegenerative disorders recently summarized the current situation as follows: "First, and most importantly, the heritability of AD is high...this had been demonstrated in various studies...over the past decades" (Bertram & Tanzi 2004: R135). These authors then go on to criticize most of the research currently being done on the genetics of AD and fault the methodology, lack of replication, and inattention to haplotype structure. Using the citation index PubMed, they show that in 2003 alone a total of 1,037 studies were done on the genetics of AD, out of which 55 analyzed genes were reported to have a positive association with increased risk for the disease, while 68 tested negative. Candidate genes were examined on every single chromosome. Bertram and Tanzi, exceedingly cautious, conclude with a caveat that "while the genetic association per se [of APOEε4 with AD] has been extremely well established over the past decade, there is no consensus as to how this association translates pathophysiologically," nor how it functions in conjunction with other numerous candidate genes (Bertram & Tanzi 2004: R137). This confusing state of affairs perhaps accounts for why, at a recent international conference on AD held in Philadelphia in 2004, the sessions that drew the biggest crowds were not those on genetics (as had been the case two years previously in Stockholm), but those on biomarkers and on mild cognitive impairment. However, there is no political economy of hope associated with this disease. A few researchers and clinicians think there will be a breakthrough in one or two years, most say five or ten, and some think we are fighting a losing battle.

TESTING FOR ALZHEIMER'S GENES

Genetic testing is routinely offered to those few people who come from families where early-onset AD is present. The basic science research on these genes is recognized as robust, and because affected individuals may have to make choices about reproductive decisions as well as prepare for the future, testing is deemed appropriate in the same way as it is for Huntington's disease (Almqvist et al. 1997; Konrad 2005).

The situation is quite different with late-onset AD. Without exception, official guidelines in North America, the United Kingdom, France, and elsewhere are at present opposed to routine testing for APOE alleles. This recommendation is easily justified, given that individual risk assessments for late-onset AD based on genotyping are at present regarded as so vague as to be deemed of little or no use in clinical care by the majority of clinicians and researchers (Farlow 1997; Liddell et al. 2001; McConnell et al. 1998; St. George-Hyslop 2000; Tilley et al. 1998). Knowledge about the genotype of a patient has absolutely no effect on clinical care or on prognosis, although it is used occasionally in support of a diagnosis of probable AD.

In reality, however, the guidelines are not always followed: Several private companies in the United States offer testing for APOE, and an Early Alert Alzheimer's Home Screening Test kit is marketed directly to consumers (Kier & Molinari 2003). At least one nursing home in North Carolina will not accept residents without first having applicants submit to an APOE test. Potential residents who test positive for APOEε4 are turned down on the grounds that they are likely to become demented and troublesome—although a case was taken to court, no settlement was reached (Thomas et al. 1998).

To date, the uptake of commercialized testing is limited. By far, the majority of APOE testing takes place in research settings where genotype analysis is routinely performed on virtually all clients and patients attending the numerous memory clinics that have mushroomed in recent years in association with neurology departments in tertiary care hospitals in North America and Europe. Patients, and in some cases their first-degree relatives, when they agree to be research subjects in connection with AD, are usually well aware that this will involve genotyping for APOE and perhaps other genes. However, these individuals are told that although genotyping is crucial for research purposes, to date knowledge about one's individual DNA has no clinical value. Consent forms make it clear that neither research subjects nor their clinicians will be given information about individual patient genotypes (although, at times, there is some slippage).

Should such testing be freed of the constraints imposed by research protocols and be introduced into clinics for routine use, as is the ultimate objective, then patients, families, and their clinicians will have to be informed about the results of DNA typing, and estimates of individual risk for AD must be discussed with them. How such risk will be calculated must inevitably be suspect, in large part because so little is understood about the epigenetics of complex disease, and the dementias are proving to be particularly stubborn in this respect. Such calculations will constitute in effect "risks that cannot be known" (Ulrich Beck, cited in Yates 2003: 96) and can hardly be counted as prescient knowledge upon which individuals or families can or should act. However, it is abundantly evident that should a medication be found that works selectively on only one of the APOE polymorphisms, as is the fervent hope of companies working on dementia pharmacogenetics, then every single patient will be tested. It is then a short step to routine testing of nonaffected relatives.

Obviously, if scientific knowledge about human molecular genomics, proteomics, and epigenetics is to make headway, particularly in connection with preventive medicine and pharmacogenetics, then researchers must procure DNA samples from thousands of volunteer subjects (it is estimated that 500 subjects and 500 controls are needed per research project; Bertram & Tanzi 2004), and, given the amount of testing that is already taking place, it is no surprise to hear from clinicians that family members of AD patients are increasingly saying that they want to be genotyped. A recent telephone survey of 314 people in the United States found that 80 percent said that if their family is predisposed to this disease, they would be willing to be genetically tested for AD if they could be reassured that the test is accurate (Neumann et al. 2001). What is more, the litigious nature of U.S. society works to encourage testing: Three lawsuits have already been brought against physicians in the United States for failing to warn family members about risks for hereditary adult-onset diseases (Offit et al. 2004).

THE REVEAL PROJECT

A National Institutes of Health (NIH) approved randomized controlled trial that goes under the name of REVEAL (Risk Evaluation and Education for Alzheimer's disease), in which volunteer subjects are tested for the APOE gene, is currently in progress. One justification for this project is to assess how people respond to being informed that they have a gene that scientists believe puts them at increased risk for late-onset Alzheimer's disease. A second is the assumption that testing for susceptibility genes is likely to become increasingly common, especially in the private sector, and therefore knowledge about how people deal with risk information when it is impossible to make predictions with a high degree of confidence is urgently needed. A third justification for REVEAL is that to withhold information from people about their bodies is patronizing, and a fourth is that in many families where someone has died of AD, members of the next generation may well believe that they have virtually a 100 percent chance of contracting the disease. If individuals can be taught, even if they are homozygous for APOEε4, that their lifetime risk for getting AD never approaches anything more than approximately 50 percent, then anxiety levels may well be lowered. The final justification for the research, and probably the most significant, is to create a pool of APOEε4 individuals whose bloods can be used at any time to "enrich clinical trials."

Families where one or more member has been affected by late-onset AD are targeted in this research, and they are recruited either through systematic ascertainment from American AD research registries kept at Boston, Case Western Reserve, and Cornell Universities, or through self-referral at each of these sites (Cupples et al. 2004). These volunteer research subjects are practicing what I characterize as corporeal citizenship, in that they believe their contribution to research will help society at large and, secondarily, possibly their own affected family member or themselves in the future.

Upon recruitment, individuals are randomized into intervention and control groups, both of which then attend a PowerPoint education session that includes information on genetic susceptibility for AD. At this point the research subjects are asked to return to the research site at a later date for a blood draw; following this, individuals in the intervention arm are informed a few weeks later about their APOE status. Subjects assigned to be controls are not given this information during the trial, even though their blood has been collected, but they eventually learn their genotype. During the course of the following twelve months, systematic monitoring of people's reactions to the project is carried out by means of three structured interviews conducted by genetic counselors. A subset of the sample, fifty-five individuals, volunteered to return after the completion of the basic REVEAL study to undergo semistructured, open-ended interviews.[5] It is of note that, on average, participants in the REVEAL project have had seventeen years of formal education, considerably higher than that for the United States as a whole.

As part of a counseling session, research subjects are provided with "personalized risk assessments" for AD in the form of graphs based on age, family history, gender, and, for those people in the experimental arm of the project, DNA typing. By the time the qualitative interviews were carried out, more than twelve months after being told of their estimated risk, participants, almost without exception, had transformed the estimates they had been given into accounts that "fit" with their ongoing experience of being related to someone with Alzheimer's disease, their individual assessment of their own family history, and the accumulated knowledge about the disease that they had gathered from a variety of sources. In other words, risk estimates given out in the REVEAL study rarely displace "popular knowledge" that participants bring with them to the project, although a small number abandon their previous belief that they will without doubt get Alzheimer's in the future. This retention of popular and personalized knowledge may in part account for the relatively small number of REVEAL participants (33 percent) who are able to accurately recall the risk estimates that they were given—particularly noteworthy when 91 percent of them stated that "wanting to know" their genotype was a major motivation for participation in the project in addition to contributing to scientific research.

GENETICS AND BLENDED INHERITANCE

Social science research has amply documented the ways in which individuals actively interpret knowledge that they are given about their genotype and frequently exhibit resistance to drawing on genetic explanations alone to account for the illnesses that "run" in their families (Condit 1999; Lock, Lloyd et al. 2006b). Furthermore, when genetic information is incorporated into accounts about illness causation, such information supplements previously held ideas about the relationship among kinship, heredity, and health. For example, Cox and McKellin (1999: 130) have demonstrated that lay understandings of heredity often conflict with theories of Mendelian genetics because scientific explanations prove to be inadequate for families dealing with the lived experience of genetic risk. Kerr et al. suggest that it is reasonable to assume that laypeople are their own authority when it comes to appreciating and understanding how genetics may shape their lives (Kerr et al. 1998).

To date, most social science research into the social ramifications of the new genetics has concentrated on the impact of transmitting information about specific genes that bring about disorders with a highly (but not 100 percent) predictable mode of Mendelian transmission. The situation is quite different when susceptibility genes are involved because estimates of risk, as noted above in the discussion of AD, are based on calculations of probability making use of variables that have low explanatory power. Adding to the complexity, professional understanding about the molecular genetics of complex disease is best described as "knowledge in flux," with the result that estimates of probability are subject to repeated revision. We are not dealing with "matters of fact" at all, but with provisional, probabilistic information that must then be translated into estimates assumed to best reflect individual cases.

If, as has been shown, professional explanations about risk in connection with Mendelian diseases do not result in the types of understanding and behaviors that have been hoped for, even when professional genetic counseling is available (Hill 1994; Rapp 1999), what might be the situation in connection with the genetics of complex diseases? Results from the REVEAL project, and from parallel research carried out in Montréal where relatives of Alzheimer patients are not genetically tested (Lock et al. 2006a), suggest that people very often draw on a concept of "blended inheritance," a form of thinking evident as early as classical times (Turney 1995: 12), when trying to interpret probability estimates given to them about their genotype. Accounts that draw on ideas about blended inheritance remain very prevalent today, and assume a mixing or blending of entities passed on from generation to generation in clusters. Phenotypic resemblances shared among family members—physical features, personality types, and so on—indicate that these same individuals are equally prone to disorders that "run in their family." It has been shown, even in connection with single-gene disorders, that this type of thinking is more common than an assumption, following Mendel, that genotype determines phenotypic expression (Richards 1996: 222). The qualitative interviews from the REVEAL study suggest, not surprisingly, that blended inheritance is made use of liberally to interpret risk estimates for AD based on APOE status and family history.

The inherent uncertainty associated with risk estimates that for by far the majority of REVEAL participants fall well below an increased risk of 50 percent by age eighty-five, compared with a "normal" population, coupled with a disease onset late in life, leaves plenty of room for research subjects to create their own personalized narratives about whether or not they are indeed vulnerable. Moreover, these individuals have an awareness, derived from the media and elsewhere (Lock, Lloyd et al. 2006), and reinforced by the REVEAL education session, that late-onset AD has multiple causes that are by no means understood, and that genetic susceptibility, although contributory, does not determine the future. Added to this is an inability on the part of some participants, despite many years of education, to effectively understand what they are being told when given information about risk and the APOE gene. Everyone who took part in REVEAL had firsthand information about what it is like to live with Alzheimer's disease, and many are also caregivers for their afflicted family member; it is this experience above all that colors responses to genotyping. For example, Carolyn, a psychiatric nurse, and her sister were both in the randomized group that received their APOE status. Carolyn learned that she has an APOEε3/3 genotype, and was told as part of the REVEAL disclosure session that she is not at high risk, whereas her sister carries a copy of the ε4 allele and was informed, therefore, that, as an APOEε3/4, she is at increased risk. When asked about her response to being tested, Carolyn says,

> In all honesty, I try not to think about it, because when I think about it I think of my sister's risk factors and—I went through it with my dad. I really don't want to think about going through it with her, you know.

When asked specifically about her reaction to her own results, Carolyn responds,

> I didn't think one way or the other when I found out my risk factor.... I guess I don't recall an awful lot.

And yet she also justifies her participation in REVEAL as having a desire to know about her genotype:

> Knowledge is power. I really believe that. I mean, I don't think you can necessarily change your destiny, but certainly to go through life with your eyes only half open doesn't help you at all.

To the question of what kinds of actions such power might motivate, Carolyn remains unsure:

> I think [REVEAL] provides useful information.... Just don't ask me how I would use it.... I honestly don't know.

During her training as a nurse, Carolyn had to complete two university courses in genetics; no doubt, this contributed to her ability to recall what she was taught in the REVEAL education session, unlike most other participants. Laura, a schoolteacher, was informed that she has a 4/4 genotype. She comments.

> I guess I thought [prior to REVEAL] I might have a 90 percent chance of having it [AD].... So, now I know my chance is fifty, fifty, so I can just say, we'll flip the coin.

> You know what, having been to, like, these little workshops, I'm still totally confused. I know I have two of them, whatever these bad things are, or something. And I've got one on my mother's side and on my father's side. So, I do know that by the time I'm, like, 70 I have a 50 percent chance of having it, which doesn't seem so bad except that most people have a 10 percent chance and reach 70. It's not too good.

When asked to explain more about the "bad things," Laura replies,

> I don't know. I don't know what gene it is.... It's not the BRCA gene.

Other people sounded equally confused, and one or two resorted to sarcasm to convey their feelings about being genotyped:

> I understand basic genetics and, you know, Mendelssohn, and those plants and stuff. I know now that APOEε4 is bad and I have one, but I don't know why it's bad or what it does. Well, I know where I am at, where I stand. I can let my kids know where we stand. You know, I mean, maybe get it, maybe not.

Several participants found that the information provided by REVEAL conflicted with their own understanding about the future. Rebecca, a 3/3 genotype with four affected relatives, insists,

> According to that [AD test], I don't have the risk, okay? So, technically I should feel better. But I don't believe it. If I had all the confidence in the world in that test, I would say: "Oh maybe it's not going to happen." But I don't think so, and even if I had a gene test come out and say: "Yes, definitively, this is you, you're going to get it," it wouldn't make any difference because I already thought I would anyway.

When asked what they think might be the cause of AD, interviewees almost without exception give multicausal explanations, although genetics is included as a contributory cause more than any other, followed by the environment, diet, and aluminum (a cause no longer subscribed to by scientists), and then numerous other variables including depression, stress, lack of mental or physical activity, and age. However, even a brief elaboration of the discussion shows at once how beliefs about genetics are embedded in complex narrative accounts. A fifty-two-year-old who was a control in the study and does not, therefore, know her APOE status reflects on matters in the following way:

> Do I think I have a higher than normal chance? Yes. Heredity. And also I'm so much like my mother. And I would say to her, "Mother, I hope I'm not like you in this regard," you know...I know that she had Alzheimer's. Fact. Therefore, there's a very high likelihood that one or more of her children will have a predisposition toward it. And I would say I'm front-runner because of so many other characteristics that are very much like my mother's.

Jane, who was given a 3/3 typing and has one affected relative, comments,

> I have—don't even know what—don't even remember because it meant so little to me.... My risk before 85 was just minimally more than others. After 85, like 15 percent more. To me, that made no sense.... I really believe I don't have much chance of missing it just by the genealogy. I mean...when I look at both sides of my family, my mother's family is all—there's nothing else, just Alzheimer's. My father's side, there's no Alzheimer's. It's heart trouble and high cholesterol and high triglycerides. Well, I take after my mother.

Another person assigned to the control group, who was unhappy that she had not been among those who were genotyped, also drew on blended inheritance to account for her concerns:

I've showed you the picture of me and my dad. We look like clones, practically, physically. And nobody's really said—I don't know whether the information is out there because I haven't read it—whether or not that makes a difference, a person's physical appearance. But I have a suspicion that it does.

One other participant comments on her brother,

My brother is very worried. He's not very sophisticated scientifically, and he tends to feel that he has inherited a lot of my mother's qualities. He has her hair color and her blue eyes and many of her behavioral traits as well. I don't mean to belittle my brother, but this is what he thinks.

Despite a strong propensity to create accounts that incorporate ideas about blended inheritance, the majority of respondents do not dwell on genetics exclusively; very frequent, too, are comments such as the following:

I think genetics plays a part, but I don't think it's the end all. I'm sure that a lot of the care about diet, and health, and the exercise that we do today will prolong life and mental acuity....

It's a kind of a Russian roulette kind of thing. Everything's got to be working against you, whatever these factors may be. And I don't even know what. Maybe aluminium in your teeth? You hear some of these things. I don't know.

Among those subjects who draw on theories of blended inheritance, a belief that biology is destiny in effect persists. This is despite participation in the REVEAL project, contrary to professional counseling and what is known about the genetics of AD, and even at times contrary to test results. On the other hand, some people apparently go away reassured that they are not at such a high risk as they had supposed, and this no doubt is a good thing, unless perhaps they are overreassured and believe that they are not after all vulnerable to the disease.

Clearly, research into endophenotypes, biomarkers, and associated susceptibility genes is crucial, but it remains an open question if it is indeed patronizing, as the justification for REVEAL suggests, to withhold from individuals the results of their genotyping, unless it is agreed by all involved that the transmission of details about what are in effect irresolvable uncertainties is of value. Interviews with REVEAL subjects indicate that tidings of uncertainty serve only to reinforce among a good number of individuals highly seductive but thoroughly outmoded beliefs, at least as far as molecular biologists are concerned, about blended inheritance. Although very few families believe that genetics are the sole cause of AD, the danger of routinizing genetic testing and informing people about their APOE status is that this practice will distract both medical experts and the public from the challenging questions raised by epigenetics, including why so many people with the ε4 polymorphism do not get AD.

Researchers and clinicians dealing with Alzheimer's disease and other dementias are fully aware of the complexity that confronts them in both the research laboratory and the clinic. At the same time, it is evident that this complexity must be scaled down if it is to become manageable. The current emphasis given to tracking down biomarkers as early signs of dementia is one clear example of this, and the continued focus on gene hunting is another. However, REVEAL researchers have carefully avoided giving their research subjects the impression that AD causality is straightforward, leaving people plenty of room for various interpretations about what their genotypes might mean for the future. It is clear that these research subjects, after learning which of the APOE polymorphisms they possess, do not come away from REVEAL questioning their identity or sense of self in any lasting way. And it seems, for the time being at least, the deeper we enter into the world of epigenetics, the less predictable will become risk estimates for complex disease based on genotyping alone. What this suggests is that the present custom of anonymizing biological materials obtained from volunteer research subjects should continue, and that these volunteers should not expect to receive personalized information about their genotype in return. Unseating the gene at center stage is not easy, but the time has come to face this challenge head-on.

NOTES

Acknowledgments. Funding for this research was provided by the Social Science and Humanities Research Council of Canada (SSHRC), grant # 205806.

The REVEAL project was supported by National Institutes of Health grants HG/AG02213 (The REVEAL Study), AG09029 (The MIRAGE Study), AG13846 (Boston University Alzheimer's Disease Center), and M01 RR00533 (Boston University General Clinical Research Center).

This article is a revised version of Margaret Lock, "La 'molécularisation' de l'esprit et la recherche sur la démence naissante," *Sciences Sociales et Santé* 24, no. 1 (March 2006): 21–56. Reprinted with kind permission from Editions John Libbey Eurotext, Paris.

1. Numerous genes are polymorphic and exhibit a number of variations that are widespread in human populations. Those polymorphisms that are associated with an increased risk for developing a disorder are known as "susceptibility genes." Such gene variants are neither necessary nor sufficient to cause specific diseases.
2. The importance of gene regulation was first noted by Jacob and Monod over forty years ago (1961), but mapping DNA structure was given priority.
3. The association between low levels of education and increased risk for late-onset AD is widely accepted as essentially verified, even though such a supposition does not fully mesh with the findings of the Nun's Study (Snowdon 2001).

4. Most current research into epigenetics focuses primarily on the expression and regulation of genes and investigates the conditions under which a gene is "switched on" or "switched off." Related questions at the phenotypic level ask why monozygotic twins do not always manifest the same diseases and, why, when they do, the age of onset can differ by up to two decades (Schmie-deskamp 2004). This narrowly conceptualized epigenetic approach makes the limitations of genetic determinism patently evident. A broader, critical form of epigenetics, known as "developmental systems theory" (DST), sup-ported by a mix of philosophers and biologists, is currently gaining ground. Using this approach, it is argued that epigenetic phenomena should be rec-ognized as having independence from genetic variation. The starting point is an ontological reversal of genetic determinism, and gives priority to dynamic interactions among very many variables with numerous possible outcomes. The biologist Scott Gilbert argues that the DST approach implies that "our 'self' becomes a permeable self. We are each a complex community, indeed, a collection of ecosystems" (Gilbert 2002: 213). At the biological level, a fun-damental question arises as to whether a gene, defined as a DNA sequence, can indeed count as the unit of heredity, especially as recent research strongly suggests that epigenetic phenomena can be transmitted from one generation to another (Champagne & Meaney 2001).

5. I was approached by one of the principal investigators of the REVEAL proj-ect to carry out the qualitative part of the research after the initial interviews were almost completed. I expressed my reservations about the project, and agreed to participate in it on the understanding that I would interview the involved clinicians and genetic counselors in addition to a sample of research subjects. Three graduate students, Janalyn Prest, Stephanie Lloyd, and Heather Lindstrom, participated in the creation of the interview protocols and carried out most of the interviews with the research subjects.

REFERENCES

Almqvist, Elisabeth, Shelin Adam, Maurice Bloch, Anne Fuller, Philip Welch, Debbie Eisenberg, Don Whelan, David Macgregor, Wendy Meschino, and Michael R. Hayden. 1997. Risk reversals in predictive testing of Huntington disease. *American Journal of Human Genetics* 61:945–52.
Angell, Marcia. 2004. The truth about the drug companies. *New York Review of Books* 51:52–58.
Armstrong, H. E. 1931. The Monds and chemical industry: A study in heredity. *Nature* 128:238.
Berg, Paul. 1991. All our collective ingenuity will be needed. *Federation of Ameri-can Societies for Experimental Biology* 5:75–77.
Bertram, Lars, and Rudolph E. Tanzi. 2004. Alzheimer's disease: One disorder, too many genes? *Human Molecular Genetics* 13, no. R1: R135–R41.
Breitner, John C. 1999. The end of Alzheimer's disease? *International Journal of Geriatric Psychiatry* 14:577–86.
Champagne, F., and M. Meaney. 2001. Like mother, like daughter: Evidence for non-genomic transmission of parental behavior and stress responsivity. *Prog-ress in Brain Research* 133:287–302.
Condit, C. M. 1999. How the public understands genetics: Non-deterministic and non-discriminatory interpretations of the "blueprint" metaphor. *Public Understanding of Science* 8:169–80.

Corbo, R. M., and R. Scacchi. 1999. Apolipoprotein E (APOE) allele distribution in the world. Is APOEε4 a 'thrifty' allele? *Ann Hum Genet* 63 (Pt 4): 301–10.

Cox, S., and W. McKellin. 1999. "There's this thing in our family": Predictive testing and the construction of risk for Huntington disease. In *Sociological perspectives on the new genetics*, edited by P. Conrad and J. Gabe. London: Blackwell.

Cupples, L. A., L. A. Farrer, A. D. Sadovnick, N. Relkin, P. Whitehouse, and R. C. Green. 2004. Estimating risk curves for first-degree relatives of patients with Alzheimer's disease: The REVEAL study. *Genetics in Medicine* 6:192–96.

Daffner, Kirk R., and Leonard F. M. Scinto. 2000. Early diagnosis of Alzheimer's disease: An introduction. In *Early diagnosis of Alzheimer's disease*, edited by L. F. M. Scinto and K. R. Daffner. Totowa, NJ: Humana Press.

Davis, B. D. 1990. The human genome and other initiatives. *Science* 4:2941–42.

DeKosky, Steven T., and Kenneth Marek. 2003. Looking backward to move forward: Early detection of neurodegenerative disorders. *Science*, 302:830–34.

Dennet, Daniel Clement. 1995. *Darwin's dangerous idea: Evolution and the meanings of life.* New York: Simon & Schuster.

Duster, Troy. 1990. *Back door to eugenics.* New York: Routledge.

Dutton, Gail. 2003. Learning the secrets of life. *Engineering News* 23:6–57.

Eddy, Sean R. 2001. Non-coding RNA genes and the modern RNA world. *Nature Reviews/Genetics* 2:919–29.

Farlow, Martin R. 1997. Alzheimer's disease: Clinical implications of the Apolipoprotein E genotype. *Neurology* 48:S30.

Fox Keller, Evelyn. 2000a. Is there an organism in this text? In *Controlling our destinies: Historical, philosophical, ethical, and theological perspectives on the HGP*, edited by P. Sloan. South Bend, IN: Notre Dame University Press.

———. 2000b. *The century of the gene.* Cambridge, MA: Harvard University Press.

———. 2002. *Making sense of life: Explaining biological development with models, metaphors and machines.* Cambridge, MA: Harvard University Press.

Gibbs, W. Wayt. 2003. The unseen genome: Gems among the junk. *Scientific American* 289, no. 5: 47–53.

Gilbert, Scott F. 2002. The genome in its ecological context: Philosophical perspectives on interspecies epigenesis. *Annals of the New York Academy of Sciences* 981:202–18.

Gottesman, I. I., and J. Shields. 1972. *Schizophrenia and genetics: A twin study vantage point.* New York: Academic Press.

Gottesman, Irving. 1994. Schizophrenia epigenesis: Past, present and future. *Acta Psychiatrica Scandinavia* 90, no. 384: S26-S33.

Grady, Denise. 2004. Nominal benefits seen in drugs for Alzheimer's. *New York Times*, April 7.

Gudding, Gabriel. 1996. The phenotype/genotype distinction and the disappearance of the body. *Journal of the History of Ideas* 57, no. 3: 525–45.

Hill, Shirley. 1994. *Managing sickle cell disease in low-income families.* Philadelphia: Temple University Press.

Jacob, François, and Jacques Monod. 1961. Genetic regulatory mechanisms in the synthesis of proteins. *Journal of Molecular Biology* 3:316–56.

Johannsen, Wilhelm. 1923. Some remarks about units in heredity. *Hereditas* 4:133–41.

Kay, Lily E. 1993. *The molecular vision of life: Caltech, the Rockefeller foundation and the new biology.* Oxford: Oxford University Press.

Kerr, A., S. Cunningham-Burley, and A. Amos. 1998. The new human genetics and health: Mobilizing lay expertise. *Public Understanding of Science* 7:41–60.

Kier, F. J., and V. Molinari. 2003. "Do-it-yourself" dementia testing: Issues regarding an Alzheimer's home screening test. *Gerontologist* 43:295–301.
Kitcher, Philip. 1996. *The lives to come: The genetics revolution and human possibilities.* New York: Simon & Schuster.
Konrad, Monica. 2005. *Narrating the new predictive genetics: Ethics, ethnography and science,* Cambridge Studies in Society and the Life Sciences, edited by N. Rose and P. Rabinow. Cambridge: University of Cambridge Press.
LeDoux, Joseph. 2002. *Synaptic self: How our brains become who we are.* London: Penguin Books.
Lewontin, Richard C. 2003. Science and simplicity. *New York Review of Books* 50, no. 7: 39–42.
Liddell, M. B., S. Lovestone, and M. J. Owen. 2001. Genetic risk of Alzheimer's disease: Advising relatives. *British Journal of Psychiatry* 178:7–11.
Lock, Margaret, Julia Freeman, Rosemary Sharples, and Stephanie Lloyd. 2006a. When it runs in the family: Putting susceptibility genes into perspective. *Public Understanding of Science* 15:277–300.
Lock, Margaret, Stephanie Lloyd, and Janalyn Prest. 2006b. Genetic susceptibility and Alzheimer's disease: The "penetrance" and uptake of genetic knowledge. In *Thinking about dementia: Culture, loss, and the anthropology of senility,* edited by A. Leibing and L. Cohen, 123–56. New Brunswick, NJ: Rutgers University Press.
Maté, Gabor. 2004. Was that trademark smile the first sign of Alzheimer's? *(London) Globe and Mail,* June 12.
Mattick, John S. 2003. Challenging the dogma: The hidden layer of non-protein-coding RNAs in complex organisms. *BioEssays* 25:930–39.
———. 2004. The hidden genetic program of complex organisms. *Scientific American* 291:60–67.
McConnell, L. M., B. A. Koenig, H. T. Greely, and A. S. Raffin. 1998. Genetic testing and Alzheimer's disease: Has the time come? *Nature Medicine* 4: 757–59.
Neumann, P. J., J. K. Hammitt, C. Muller, H. M. Fillit, J. Hill, N. A. Tetteh, and K. S. Kosik. 2001. Public attitudes about genetic testing for Alzheimer's disease. *Health Affairs* 20, no. 5: 252–64.
Novas, Carlos, and Nikolas Rose. 2000. Genetic risk and the birth of the somatic individual. *Economy and Society* 29:485–513.
Offit, Kenneth, Elizabeth Groeger, Sam Turner, Eve A. Wadsworth, and Mary A. Weiser. 2004. The "duty to warn" a patient's family member about heredity disease risks. *Journal of the American Medical Association* 292:1469–73.
Petronis, Arturas. 2001. Human morbid genetics revisited: Relevance of epigenetics. *Trends in Genetics* 17:142–46.
Pritchard, C., D. Baldwin, and A. Mayers. 2004. Changing patterns of adult (45–74 years) neurological deaths in the major Western countries 1979–1997. *Public Health* 118:268–83.
Rapp, Rayna. 1999. *Testing women, testing the fetus: The social impact of amniocentesis in America.* New York: Routledge.
Rheinberger, Hans-Jörg. 1995. From microsomes to ribosomes: "Strategies" of "Representation" 1935–1955. *Journal of the History of Biology* 28:49–89.
Richards, Martin. 1996. Lay and professional knowledge of genetics and inheritance. *Public Understanding of Science* 5:217–30.
Sapp, Jan. 1983. The struggle for authority in the field of heredity, 1900–1932: New perspectives on the rise of genetics. *Journal of the History of Biology* 16, no. 3: 311–42.

Schmiedeskamp, Mia. 2004. Preventing good brains from going bad. *Scientific American* 14:84–91.

Scinto, Leonard F., and Kirk R. Daffner, eds. 2000. *Early Diagnosis of Alzheimer's Disease*. Totawa, NJ: Humana Press.

Selkoe, Dennis J. 2002. The Pathophysiology of Alzheimer's Disease. In *Early Diagnosis of Alzheimer's Disease*. L. F. M. Scinto and K. R. Daffner, eds. Totawa, NJ: Humana Press.

Silver, M. H., K. Newell, E. T. Hedley-White, and T. T. Perls. 2001. Distinguishing between neurodegenerative disease and disease-free aging: Correlating neuropsychological evaluations and neuropathological studies in centenarians. *Psychosomatic Medicine* 64:493–501.

Snowdon, David. 2001. *Aging with grace: What the nun study teaches us about leading longer, healthier, and more meaningful lives*. New York: Bantam Books.

Stafford, Philip B. 1991. The social construction of Alzheimer's Disease. In *Biosemiotics: The Semiotic Web*, edited by Thomas A. Sebeok and Jean Umiker-Sebeok, 393–406. Berlin: Mouton de Gruyter.

St. George-Hyslop, P. H. 2000. Molecular genetics of Alzheimer's disease. *Biological Psychiatry* 47:183–99.

Swartz, R. H., S. E. Black, and P. St. George-Hyslop. 1999. ApolipoproteinE and Alzheimer's disease: A genetic, molecular and neuroimaging review. *Canadian Journal of Neurological Sciences* 26:77–88.

Thomas, A. Mathew, Gene Cohen, Robert M. Cook-Deegan, Joan O'Sullivan, Stephen G. Post, Allen D. Roses, Kennneth F. Schaffner, and Ronald M. Green. 1998. Alzheimer testing at silver years. *Cambridge Quarterly of Healthcare Ethics* 7:294–307.

Tilley, L., K. Morgan, and N. Kalsheker. 1998. Genetic risk factors in Alzheimer's disease. *Journal of Clinical Pathology: Molecular Pathology* 51:293–304.

Turney, Jon. 1995. The public understanding of genetics—Where next? *European Journal of Genetics and Society* 1:5–22.

Watson, James, and Francis Crick. 1953. The structure of DNA. *Cold Spring Harbor Symposia on Quantitative Biology* 18:123–31.

Whitehouse, Peter J. 2001. The end of Alzheimer disease. *Alzheimer Disease and Associated Disorders* 15, no. 2: 59–62.

Yates, Joshua. 2003. An interview with Ulrich Beck on fear and risk society. *Hedgehog Review* 5:96–107.

5 Embodied action, enacted bodies
The example of hypoglycaemia

Annemarie Mol and John Law

LIVING BODIES

We all know this: that the living body is both an object and a subject.

We know that the body is an *object* of medical knowledge. When it is observed with the naked eye and through microscopes, CT scans and other visual machinery the body is an object. It is an object when it is measured in a variety of ways, from counting the pulse to determining the blood levels of haemoglobin, creatinin, calcium. And the body-object may be sensed as well: when the hands of the doctor feel for lumps, or for points of orientation in an operation.

The living body is a *subject,* too. It is us, we: for it is as embodied that we are human beings. So the body is the fleshy condition for, or, better, the fleshy situatedness of, our modes of living. In being a living body we experience pain, hunger, or agony as well as satisfaction, ecstasy, or pleasure. And while the object-body is exposed and publicly displayed, the subject-body is private and beyond, or before, language.

If one wants to write about living bodies this seems to be the place to start, this *given*, that we have a public body-object and *are* a private subject-body. It has been articulated in philosophy, anthropology, and sociology as well as in medicine.[1] It appears time and again in testimonies of real life experience. It is what we all know. But maybe it is time to escape from this self-evidence. Maybe it is time to start knowing something else—or in another way.

The body has not always been an object/subject. Michel Foucault suggests that this is a *trope* that was invented in the early nineteenth century (Foucault 1976). Before then, diseases were entities in their own right, classified in nosological tables. Patients seeking relief would describe the ailments they were suffering from, and doctors would then infer which disease was *inhabiting* the patient's body—and what might next happen. A radical epistemic shift was needed for diseases to become conditions of the human body. After this shift the truth about a disease could no longer be detected by listening to the patient's words. Instead it required a well-trained gaze at bodily tissues. Since deviant tissues are usually hidden beneath the skin, sure knowledge about diseases could only be established after death. So the body-object/subject-body distinction with which we now live was established. In the words of Mark Sullivan:

> For Bichat, the medical subject and the medical object were not two different substances within the same individual, but two different individuals: one alive and one dead. Knower and known are epistemologically distinguished with the physician assuming the position of the knower and the patient/corpse the position of the known. (Sullivan 1986: 344)

Sullivan argues that this split generates the crucial dualism that troubles modern medicine. This is not the dualism attributed to Descartes, between two kinds of substance, body and mind; instead it is the distinction between substance and activity:

> Here, the activity of self-interpretation or self-knowledge is eliminated from the body rather than the entity of mental substance. The body known and healed by modern medicine is not self-aware. (Sullivan 1986: 344)

Sullivan and many others seek to integrate people's self-awareness back into modern medicine.[2] But how? Most authors suggest addition: alongside, or on top of, pathological knowledge of tissues and their deviances, doctors should make space for the self-awareness of their patients. They want medicine not only to look but also to listen; to grant patients their life as well as knowing them as if they were dead.

Although it may seem hard to disagree with Sullivan's plea for a medicine that attends not only to its patients' organs but also to their self-awareness, there is the problem that it leaves untouched the modes of knowing involved. On the one hand there is an objective, public, and scientific way of knowing the body from the outside. On the other hand there is a subjective, private, and personal way of knowing the body from the inside. These are the modes of knowing invented in Bichat's time. Foucault describes how the modern epistème (of which they form a part) is linked up with the *birth of the clinic*. Modern medicine and the gaze at dead and deviant tissues came into being with a specific kind of hospital, a specific system for medical training, and a specific set of practices for treatment. Together they gave pathology the last word, while a wide range of techniques (from X-ray to laboratory chemistry) were developed to look beneath the skin of living bodies. And it was only with this way of ordering medical knowledge that the self-awareness of patients was privatised.[3]

Since quite a lot of time has passed since the early nineteenth century we would like to use Foucault's work not as a finished description of "modernity" but as an inspiration for asking whether we still live within the same modern episteme. We would like to ask about the modes of knowing exhibited in current medical practices, about how the body is currently known. But to put it in this way is already too restrictive because it assumes that it is *knowledge* that is central. In order to evade this assumption it may be more promising to ask a slightly different question: what is a body in the conditions of possibility at the beginning of the twenty-first century? To phrase it in this way is risky. The danger is that the answer will simply repeat what has already been said by biomedical experts or patients: hardly a real contribution. Seeking to add to or correct the knowledge of experts or patients with only the techniques of ethnography at our disposal would be equally futile. No, we don't "know better." Asking the question "what *is* a body" is worthwhile in quite a different way. It is a way of shifting the grounds on which questions about the reality of bodies may be posed. It moves us to a place where gathering *knowledge*—whether objective or subjective—is no longer idolized as the most important way of relating to and being in the world.

We all *have* and *are* a body. But there is a way out of this dichotomous twosome. As part of our daily practices, we also do (our) bodies. In practice we enact them. If the body we *have* is the one known by pathologists after our death, while the body we *are* is the one we know ourselves by being self-aware, then what about the body we *do*? What can be found out and said about it? Is it possible to inquire into the body we *do*? And what are the consequences if action is privileged over knowledge? In order to explore this we will tell you some stories about hypoglycaemia taken from a continuing study of living with diabetes.[4]

KNOWING HYPOGLYCAEMIA IN PRACTICE

So what is hypoglycaemia? This comes from a medical textbook:[5]

> In people without diabetes mellitus plasmaglucose levels vary between 3 and 8 mmol/l, depending on the time that has passed since the last meal. In general the criterion for hypoglycaemia in a patient with diabetes is set at a blood glucose level under 3.5 mmol/l. (van Haeften 1995: 142)

In this definition hypoglycaemia is located *beneath the skin* and is a characteristic state of a mobile bodily tissue, blood. It is a blood glucose level below 3.5 mmol/l. This, then, is an object-definition in line with the tradition of pathology, portraying a body-we-have. But the textbook locates hypoglycaemia in other places too: "Hypoglycaemia is a frequently occurring, potentially serious complication in the treatment of diabetes mellitus." (idem)

The treatment of diabetes mellitus is not located *in* the body but in hospitals, information leaflets, and people's homes. It is in the *daily lives* of people who suffer from diabetes mellitus. In daily life hypoglycaemia is something that may occur, happen, be done. It is a potentially serious complication.

It is easy to find sentences like this in medical textbooks and scientific articles: sentences in which phenomena are presented as being part of the practices in which they occur.[6] But not just anywhere. Practicalities tend to appear in the *materials and methods* section of papers but not in the conclusions. They tend to appear in clinical presentations but not in epidemiological overviews. Knowledge about a body-we-have and knowledge about a body-we-do tend to alternate. So the shift we are proposing is quite simple even though it has far-reaching consequences. It is to keep the practicalities in the foreground the whole time. Never taking the short-cut of understanding "hypoglycaemia" as hidden *in* the body or beneath the skin, our ethnographic description consistently attends to the practices in which it is being done.

So *how* is hypoglycaemia done? A first important mode is, indeed, by *knowing* it. Knowing is a practice: it only becomes possible to talk about "a blood sugar level below 3.5 mmol/l" if someone's skin is pricked, a blood sample is taken, and its sugar level is measured. This used to happen in the laboratory. A technician would puncture a vein, collect some blood in a small tube, insert it in a machine, and read the outcome. This still happens, but it has been joined by another measurement practice. Since the necessary machinery has been miniaturised, people with diabetes can now carry it round with them and measure their own blood sugar levels. They prick a finger tip and squeeze a drop of blood onto a measurement stick. The stick is put into a slot in the machine and within a few seconds a number is displayed. However, none of this is easy: Pricking the finger may hurt, the number may take some while to appear, and so on. Measurement is demanding and sometimes impossible to handle in practice. Here is an internist in an interview:

> I understand perfectly well it isn't always easy. Like this patient I have who works on the roads. You sit there, in a ditch, dirt all round you, your hands are filthy, nowhere to hide. I wouldn't measure either, if I were in his position.

Dirty ditches are a problem. But measuring your blood sugar level is also difficult in a management meeting where you cannot withdraw for a minute or two, or if you are shopping in town with your friends; or if you are teaching a class of children. Nevertheless, it is possible to measure one's blood sugar level in a clean kitchen or in the bathroom—that is, in a location in which circumstances are as well tamed as in a laboratory. In this way hypoglycaemia may be *enacted* as a blood sugar level below 3.5 mmol/l.

Sullivan and many other critics argue that medicine should know living bodies in a way that is richer than the knowledge of silenced corpses. It should appreciate that patients are able to act. But asking people with diabetes to be active as laboratory technicians doesn't do the trick: it merely turns them into their own pathologists. It does not do away with the dualism between the knowing doctor and the patient whose body is known but simply shifts this, so that it starts to run right through every individual. Attending not only to the body we *have* but also the body we *are* requires knowledge from the inside. And interestingly, in the day-to-day handling (or avoiding) of hypoglycaemia, *self-awareness* is at least as important as measuring. For if one is sensitive to one's own physical state from the inside, one can feel a hypoglycaemia (a "hypo") coming on, and do something to increase one's blood sugar level. But being self-aware is not self-evident. It is not something that all people are able to do so long as medicine is not silencing them. Some people are good at it, others are not. As a diabetes nurse puts it:

> Sometimes we have people here who never feel anything. They just do what's on their list. So you try to give them a good list, tell them what to do when, and put some extra measurement moments in. But then when something unexpected happens, they run into problems. While others, well, they tell me they hardly ever measure apart from one or two control days, but they never report any hypos either. They somehow seem to feel it coming.

The diabetes nurse believes that people who "somehow seem to feel it coming" are better off because they can lead more flexible lives. They can deal with an unexpected hypoglycaemia that may occur if they have departed from their routines. She enthusiastically describes how she participates in programmes of group instruction where self-awareness is being taught to those who lack it.[7] In the treatment of people with diabetes, then, self-awareness is not silenced by medicine, but used as a resource—and extended where this is possible.[8]

There may be a dualism between knowing bodies objectively from the outside or subjectively from the inside. But if, as we are suggesting, practice is persistently foregrounded, then it appears that the relation between measuring and "intro-sensing" hypoglycaemia is more complex. Sometimes, and for some people, feeling bad is enough of a reason to act. Measuring is simply unnecessary. But in other circumstances intro-sensing and measuring are thrown into contrast and the latter is advertised as being more accurate. This is because feeling bad does not necessarily relate to a hypo, but may also be the effect of a drop in blood sugar level from, say, 15 to 8 mmol/l. This means that feeling bad isn't necessarily a reason for increasing one's blood sugar level, but should instead be a reason for measuring it. And some people don't "feel bad" at all, so they may always have to measure if they want to assess their blood sugar level. But from the ethnographer's point of view the most interesting relation between objectivity and subjectivity comes with the use of measurement machines to train inner sensitivity. In training programmes people are told to guess their blood sugar levels first, before they measure them. The object is not to turn them into accurate number-guessers, but to encourage them to stop whatever they are doing in order to feel their bodies from inside. It is to seduce them into practicing self-awareness.

COUNTERACTING, AVOIDING, PRODUCING HYPOGLYCAEMIA

But doing hypoglycaemia is not only a matter of knowing it by measuring it from the outside, feeling it from the inside, or some combination of the two. Miriam T has lived with diabetes for years. When we asked her "What is hypoglycaemia?" she told a different story:

> Well if at the moment that we diabetics go to sleep we have [a blood sugar of] 4 [mmol/], then you simply know that at some point you run a risk of getting a hypo in the night, that it's too low. It should be 6 or 7, but what happens is that, well, oh, shit, I wake up in the middle of the night and shiver, shiver, shiver, and sweat, and then I have to get out of bed and eat something. Not if I'm being well-behaved, but if I'm careless, well, yes, then I have to get out of bed.

In this story there are numbers (4, 6, 7) and there is shivering and sweating. But Miriam T. also talks about getting up in the middle of the night, angry with herself for having been careless. The crucial action required is that of eating.

> And then I scold myself and go to the fridge, I take out the yoghurt and put some sugar in it. And sometimes I sit there on the floor, eating, for that's all I can do at a moment like that, sit on the cold floor of the kitchen and eat my yoghurt with sugar. And then gradually I get better.

In the daily lives of people with diabetes hypoglycaemia is something they know about, but the point of their dealings with it is not to gather knowledge but to intervene. For Miriam T. the most interesting way of relating to hypoglycaemia is neither to feel nor to measure but to *counteract* it. So when asked what a hypoglycaemia is, she talks about getting up in the night and eating sugary yoghurt.[9] Some people even do hypoglycaemia without ever getting to know it at all. They try to avoid it at all costs. As a diabetes nurse reports:

We also have this patient, an elderly woman who got insulin-dependent recently, who is so afraid of getting a hypo that whenever she feels bad, she eats. So she eats and eats. And she doesn't like to measure her own blood sugar, so she may feel bad, not because her blood sugar is low, but simply because it has just dropped. It was, say, 15 and it dropped to 8 and that makes her feel bad and she wants to avoid having a hypo and she eats—and eats till her sugar is 15 again. And then she"s miserable because, you know, she's getting fat.

Being fat is not a "clinical sign" of hypoglycaemia and yet it may be part of a specific mode of enacting it, that of *avoidance*. Avoiding hypoglycae-mia by eating whenever one feels bad is not a course of action encouraged by nurses. However, it is comprehensible, for there are good reasons for avoiding hypoglycaemia. Here's Miriam T. again: "With insulin, after all, you have a lethal drug in the house. People get killed with it. If you shoot up too much and eat nothing, well, then you die."

In current treatment practices people with diabetes learn to inject their own insulin, but not too much of it. They learn to counteract hypogly-caemia, or, preferably, to prevent it from occurring at all, not by eating whenever they feel bad, but only when this is really necessary. Measuring and feeling form only a small part of all the activities required of "active patients," and acquiring knowledge is not the aim of these activities. Bal-ancing food intake, exercise, and insulin injections, people with diabetes try, instead, to avoid hypoglycaemias—and hyperglycaemias, too. They must maintain their blood sugar levels at a *proper target level*.

Medicine has changed these target levels over the last couple of decades. Ideal blood sugar levels are now lower than they used to be, since holding them low tends to postpone the onset of secondary complications. These complications are nasty: as people with diabetes get older they are more likely than others to go blind, to suffer from neuropathy, or to develop ath-erosclerosis. In clinical trials there have been comparisons between people treated in the traditional way (with a single insulin injection a day and a three-monthly laboratory control measurement of average blood sugar level) and those whose blood sugar levels were tightly regulated at lower levels (maintained with several smaller daily insulin injections and as many self-administered blood sugar measurements as necessary). The second group turned out to have a better statistical chance of long term health. As one internist says:

Twelve, fifteen years ago you could still have done a proper trial to investigate whether tight regulation really improves patients' long term outcomes. But now this wouldn't be ethical. You no longer can. Enough proof has been assembled, even though the trials that were done didn't all follow what I think are good treatment programs.

The current treatment policy is one of tight regulation wherever possible. Statistically this improves people's long-term state of health, but it has the disadvantage that it leads to a higher incidence of hypoglycaemia. If target levels are set lower it is not surprising that the frequency of blood sugar levels that are too low increases. Thus, while individuals are taught to avoid hypoglycaemias and to counteract them as quickly as possible, recent clinical trials—and the standards that have followed from them—actively produce hypoglycaemia. This, of course, is not something that has been sought after, but is a negative trade-off of postponing long-term complications. It turns out, then, that medical practice is not primarily interested in knowing hypoglycaemia either. In clinical encounters professionals try to increase their patients' ability to avoid or counteract hypoglycaemia, while implementing state-of-the art treatment programmes causes the overall increase in "hypoglycaemic incidents"—as a *side-effect*.

IN- AND EXCORPORATIONS

We asked "what is hypoglycaemia" and have found that it may be: measured as a blood sugar level below 3.5 mmol/; felt as sweating, shivering, or an overall sense of discomfort; countered as something that responds to eating sugar; avoided out of fear of coma or, worse, death; while it is also produced as a negative trade-off of postponing long-term complications. Done in all these ways, hypoglycaemia is all these things.[10] But what do they imply for the body? The answer is, two things: First, as they enact hypoglycaemia, bodies *do* a lot of things: they *act*. And second, while it is measuring, feeling, countering, avoiding, and producing hypoglycaemia the body is *being enacted*, too. But no, it is more complicated still: for acting and being enacted go together. Thus we may ask: while it is acting, what is a body made to be? This is the question to which we now turn.

Pathologists who observe corpses, or doctors who use instruments in order to see through the skin of a living patient, are primarily concerned with watching. This, at any rate, is the way in which Foucault described the "clinical gaze," the dominant medical mode of knowing that came into being in the early nineteenth century. The doctor's body is active in the gaze, but only partially. It is primarily the eyes that do the gazing. The technologies that help the physician to "see through" the skin of living bodies may also address the ears, or the observer's sense of touch or even smell—even if the dominant knowledge-metaphor remains visual.[11] When Sullivan and others ask us to appreciate the self-awareness of the patient they are stressing the importance of another sensory faculty: that of feeling the degree of physical well-being from the inside. Thus the knowledge of bodies involves all the senses,[12] and knowledge-in-practice involves yet more of the body—such as hands that have to manipulate and should not shake too much. Other ways of enacting hypoglycaemia depend not only on the hands, but also on the biting mouth, the digesting intestines, and the sugar metabolism of each individual cell. Enacting hypoglycaemia involves the whole body. But this body is not a well-defined whole: it is not closed off, but has semi-permeable boundaries.

Let us start with measuring. This certainly depends on the eyes that have to read the display on the measurement machine. But before the eyes the hands have been active. They prick and are pricked. Aim well, next to the fingertip but not in it: if you happen to go blind later in life you will need your fingertips to feel your way round. One hand squeezes a drop of blood out of the other. The hands, too, insert the stick that has absorbed the blood into the slot in the measurement machine—so long as all goes well. The diabetes nurse:

> Sometimes I don't understand industry. Here, try, can you open the cap of this bottle? I can hardly do it myself. And a lot of people with diabetes, when they get older, they have more trouble using their hands. Or, with old people, their hands tremble too much for them to insert a stick into a slot, here, look, this machine here, impossible! Then there are machines around with displays so small that the numbers are hardly readable at all, let alone for someone with bad eyes. But then again, something big and solid that everybody could use, young people don't like that. They want something they can carry everywhere, something small. Fashionably designed, too, so that they can show it off.

Hands are active in measuring hypoglycaemia but they do not act alone. They interact with machinery. The success of this interaction depends on the extent to which hands and machines are adapted and adaptable to one another. Some things can be done, if only a body is prepared and trained to do them—others falter when a machine is not properly adjusted to the body it must serve. Machines only become instruments if the body can manipulate them and incorporate them in its actions,[13] so measuring depends on an open rather than an isolated body. The actively measuring body merges with its measurement machines. What about the body that feels? Miriam T., in the middle of the interview: "Well, excuse me. I've got to go to the kitchen now, I must eat an apple or something."

Miriam T. feels a hypoglycaemia coming on and fetches an apple—or something—in order to counteract it. She doesn't measure her blood sugar level: she dislikes pricking her finger and avoids doing it if she can.[14] But neither does her feeling derive from an isolated and well-bounded body: it includes a lot more.

> Me, well, I know my body pretty well, and if I were to prick and measure myself right now, I know that I'm fairly low, for I feel kind of, eh, I've got to eat something extra, because I've injected too much. That is, we were having chili tonight and that's with beans and that's a lot

of carbohydrates, and then I tend to inject two or three units more so that it doesn't go up too much, but now I've been doing things in the garden, so, hmm, I have to eat an extra something because otherwise I won't do well. But now we can have nuts in a bit, so I do allow myself that, hah, nuts.

In her appreciation of herself as being "low," Miriam T. includes: carbohydrate tables and her experience with measurement machines; the chili she has eaten; the units of insulin she has injected; her gardening; and even the promise of nuts. She incorporates what surrounds her. The self-aware body has semi-permeable boundaries. But not only does what was outside the body come inside, but there is also movement in the other direction. Some bodily activities may take place beyond the surface of the skin. Miriam T.'s husband Josef, for instance, happens to be very good at detecting Miriam T.'s hypoglycaemias:

> Then he looks at me and says "Don't you think you'd better eat something?" Or he doesn't even look, but he gets it from how I'm doing. I get irritated in a particular way, or unfriendly. And he knows where I'm at, what's happening. And usually he's right.

Later Josef came into the room and admitted with some pride that he could often feel when Miriam T. was becoming unwell. Indeed, he did not talk about *seeing* but about *feeling* it. Thus, while a body-in-practice may incorporate some of its surroundings it may also, how to say this, excorporate some of its actions. The very activity of intro-sensing may take place outside one's body-proper.

Physical action is needed in measuring and feeling, but also in counteracting hypoglycaemia. To do something about feeling "low" Miriam T. must bite, chew, and swallow. She must do this for herself: no one else can do it for her. But she cannot do it by herself. She needs an apple—or something—to eat. If people are to counteract a hypoglycaemia physically, their surroundings must be prepared for action. Miriam T:

> I never leave the house without food in my bag. Never. Without insulin in my bag, without dextrose in my bag, never. No matter what, I've always got my bag with me. For when I am somewhere, standing somewhere, and have to eat something, well, then I can't have that, that I have nothing with me.

Miriam takes food whenever she goes somewhere, and has carefully spread dextrose and biscuits around. They are in the glove compartment of her car, in the panniers on her bicycle, in the bedroom upstairs. "That has become ordinary, it belongs to me. That is me."

We just put it like this: in addition to one's body, one's surroundings have to be ready for action. But we may also follow Miriam T.'s suggestion: well-prepared surroundings become part of the active self, *me*, which means that this is far larger than the body.

In enacting hypoglycaemia, bodies act. But these active bodies are not isolated. Instead their boundaries are leaky. They interact and sometimes partially merge with their surroundings. This is even more obvious when measuring and feeling are forgotten, and action comes too late. For if a hypoglycaemia becomes really bad the body begins to lose its capability of acting properly all by itself. With a blood sugar level that is very low one starts to behave strangely, aggressively, as if drunk. Miriam T. has warned her colleagues.

> So I've said to them, if I'm ever in a state like that, take me out of the main part of the shop, take me out of the shop to the stock room or the office, wherever, the toilets, I don't care, but I would feel embarrassed if I'd been having a good hypo in the shop.

A severe hypoglycaemia is seriously incapacitating. First the body becomes untrustworthy and embarrassing; later it may slide into a coma. In a coma one cannot eat or drink even if sugar is available. Instead an injection of glucagon is needed: the hormone that leads the body to release part of its store of sugar into the bloodstream. A comatose body can still respond to glucagon, but someone else needs to do the injecting. Josef and a few of Miriam T's colleagues in the supermarket have learned how to do this. If her hands and mouth are no longer able to act it is they who must counteract her hypoglycaemias. Here again, then, as with measuring and feeling, the boundaries of the body-in-practice are partially permeable. An active body incorporates bits and pieces of the world around it, while its action may be shifted out of the body, excorporated.

Persistently foregrounding practice changes our appreciation of the body, the body-in-action. Observing eyes are still important (they must read the numbers on the display of the measurement machine) but they are joined by manipulating hands (which prick and squeeze out blood, or carry sugar to the mouth). Intro-sensing remains important, but eating and drinking appear to be even more crucial to survival. Indeed, the paradigmatic activity of the body-in-action is not observation, but metabolization. This suggestion fits well with our earlier observation that the active body has semi-permeable boundaries. An observing body does not: it sees what is outside, and feels what is within. Our eyes look around, while one of the crucial steps in acquiring self-awareness is the ability to differentiate between self and other, between who one is from the inside and what, being outside it, one is not.[15] However, for the metabolic body, inside and outside are not so stable. Metabolism, after all, is about eating, drinking, and breathing; about defecating, urinating, and sweating. For a metabolic body incorporation and excorporation are essential.

NON/COHERENCES

The body is actively engaged in enacting hypoglycaemia; (the threat of) hypoglycaemia, in its turn, helps to enact the body—in a quite specific way. There are many different ways of enacting bodies.[16] For instance, living with asthma makes people acutely aware of the air they breathe, as does practicing yoga (Willems 1998). People who have gone blind later in life have given gripping descriptions of the opaque, obstacle-ridden space they have come to inhabit (Golledge 1997). Transsexuality comes with an overwhelming sense of living in a sexed body with genitals that are either inappropriate or desirable (Hirschauer 1993). The gym may produce strong muscles or give one a sense of their inadequacy. Those who try to lose weight come to inhabit a metabolic reality in which food consists of calories, and physical exercise is a way to lose these. And, returning to the day-to-day reality of living with diabetes, here the body is also enacted as a metabolic system, though now appreciating food is matter of calculating carbohydrates and doing exercise a way of burning sugar. What is primarily at stake is short term sugar balance rather than long term accumulation of body fat.

In the metabolic system relevant to living with diabetes many things are linked together: food with insulin with exercise with blood sugar level. Blood sugar level, in its turn, has yet more physical links, since over time high blood sugars cause arterial obstruction by atherosclerosis, a deterioration of eyesight, and a loss of sensitivity due to degradation of the neurons. The body is entangled in ever so many ways with the diabetes it lives with. And yet it is not a coherent whole. Instead, it is a set of tensions. For instance, there are tensions between the interests of its various organs. Regulating blood sugar tightly may be good for the arteries, the eyes, and the neurons, but since it increases the risk of hypoglycaemia, it is bad for the brain. Internist:

> Let me tell you, it worries me, it does. Since these trials have been published tight regulation has become too popular. My younger colleagues tend to go for it, just like that, without wondering if people are really up to it, if they can stay low without sliding into too many hypos. It is in the literature, it is "science based!" The less experience doctors have the more they love the "science based." But we've started to ask patients a bit more systematically about their hypoglycaemic incidents, making them keep diaries and stuff, and the numbers they report are shocking, a lot higher than we estimated. And I've looked into the literature a bit, for gradually there's more research into hypoglycaemia of

course, and there is one report after another about hypos causing brain damage. Nobody knows just yet how much brain damage.

Tight regulation is not good or bad for the body as a whole. It is good for some parts of the body and bad for others. Thus there are tensions, in both the body and people's daily lives. What is the least bad option: To allow a higher blood sugar level and risk atherosclerosis, blindness, or lack of neuronal sensitivity in twenty years? Or to hold it lower, but to risk hypoglycaemias that straight away mean that it is dangerous to drive or carry children because of the possibility of coma? Which life to live, and which body: A body that loses count and has shaking hands but can feel? Or a body with clogged arteries that has gone blind and can't feel too well, but at least is clearheaded? Such are the options which confront people with diabetes (Mol 1998).

But no, it is misleading to talk about options. For if one had a choice it would be obvious what to opt for: an ideally balanced combination—tight regulation, a low blood sugar level, and the quick detecting and countering of hypoglycaemias. This ideal, however, is unsustainable. It depends on the ability to assess one's blood sugar level, calculate what one eats, and keep track of the energy one uses up in exercise—unremittingly, moment by moment, without ever stopping. But there is more. The most tantalizing feature of trying to maintain a stable blood sugar balance is that one may still fail, however hard one tries. Sometimes blood sugars simply behave in unpredictable ways. Miriam T.:

> You never know what's done it. Emotions are typically hard to deal with, very much so. They may be energy spenders, paff, there you go, a bit of laughing or crying, and you have a low. But then again: they may also lead to the release of whatever sugar you store. Then when I do a measurement I think: I didn't eat anything for hours. So why is it thirteen, thirteen?

Sugar balance is part of a metabolic system: the term suggests a closed circuit, but some variables are always missing. They behave unpredictably or they are not known. This means that the obligation of constant control implies the threat of unexpected failure. And you never know what's done it. The same is true for long-term complications. Low blood sugar targets are intended to prevent secondary complications, but even those who follow a tight regime may still fall victim to them. Internist:

> And then people say to me, they say: "Oh, doctor, I saw this person in the waiting room, and one of his legs had been amputated. That scares me, it scares the hell out of me. Now if I do my self-controls properly, and stay below ten as I should, please promise me that it won't happen to me, that I'll have to have a leg amputated." That's what they want

to be reassured about. But of course I can't promise anything. I wish I could, but I can't.

Statistically the correlations are clear: tightly regulated blood sugar balances lead to fewer complications later in life than blood sugar levels that are high or jump up and down. But what happens to individuals is unpredictable. Eyes go blind, or they do not. The development of neuropathy may be postponed, or not. Atherosclerosis may develop quickly, or not—and if it develops quickly the leg arteries may deteriorate so much that amputation is the only way to stop pain, or prevent gangrene and death. This, then, is a second tension that plagues the body living with diabetes: the tension between control and capriciousness. However many calculations one makes, one's blood sugar level will still behave erratically. However successfully one's life may be under control, it still throws up distressing surprises. Modern diabetes treatment demands that patients consistently keep accounts of everything about their bodies, even if it appears in the process that those bodies cannot be counted on.

A third tension arises from the way in which a variety of necessities and aspirations have to be held together and embodied, as we might put it, "single-bodiedly." The body-with-diabetes comes with a set of tensions, but people with diabetes are not only "people with diabetes." They may have asthma, do yoga, be blind or transsexual, go to the gym, or try to lose weight. They may work in ditches, at board meetings, or in front of classrooms. They may fall in love or out of it, have depressions or attacks of flu, go on holiday, work in the garden, go shopping or take exams. The specificities of the other ways in which people live their bodies somehow have to be combined with those to do with diabetes.

> Cecilia H.: I was a real sports person. I loved to run, swim, cycle, play volleyball, tennis, lots of things. So that is what I was most concerned about when I heard about my diagnosis, that I would have to give up that part of me. And at first, indeed, I felt so miserable I thought I'd feel weak as water for the rest of my life. But then gradually I've conquered it, got it back, sport, quite a lot of it really. I simply wanted it. I wanted it so much. And I did it. But it wasn't easy, it still isn't. For the point is: you may get a hypo when your muscles use up so much energy, not just then and there, immediately, but even hours and hours later. So if you run in the afternoon, you risk a hypo in the night.

The body of the sports person and the body of the person-with-diabetes are in tension. The bursts of energy of the former do not coexist very well with the precarious energy balance of the latter. This is a difficult tension. Some people successfully manage the ceaseless business of juggling it, and live with it for a long time. Those who cannot do this have to give up "a part of themselves." If dealing with hypos that come in the night is too complicated, they may give up being a sports person. But if they stick to sport and test the limits then there is the risk that one day they fall over the edge and die.[17] What this suggests is that the assumption that we have a coherent body or are a whole hides a lot of work. This is work someone has to do. You do not have, you are not, a body-that-hangs-together, naturally, all by itself. Keeping yourself whole is one the tasks of life. It is not given but must be achieved, both beneath the skin and beyond, in practice.

WHAT FOLLOWS

In the Western theoretical tradition "the body" is characteristically evoked as the exemplary case of what it is to be whole. An "organic whole" may even sound like a tautology.[18] This fits with knowing the body as something we have and something we are. The body-we-have, awaiting the gaze of the observer on the examination table, does not extend beyond the edges of the table. It stays passively within its skin. The observer's task is to understand how it hangs together: the systematic coherence of the body-we-have is never questioned. But the body-we-are is also, or should be, a whole. People whose body-images are not coherent, who do not feel their bodies to be integrated, are diagnosed as deviant. And modern medicine, with its plurality of specialties, is widely criticized for failing to appreciate our wholeness. If we are a whole, or so the criticism goes, why are we not treated accordingly?

However, if we foreground the practices for dealing with reality and do so persistently, the body's "organic wholeness" is no longer self-evident. But this does not imply that the body we do is fragmented, the converse of being whole. If we were to do our bodies in ways that fragmented them, death would quickly follow. The body we do is neither a whole, nor fragmented; instead it has a complex configuration.[19] There are boundaries around the body we do: it is Miriam T. who shivers when she has a hypo in the night and not Joseph, her husband. But these boundaries are semi-permeable: Joseph may feel Miriam T.'s hypo for her, and the sweet yoghurt she eats stops her hypo. So long as it does not disintegrate, the body-we-do hangs together. It is, however, full of tensions. There are tensions between the interests of its various organs. There are tensions between taking control and being erratic. There are tensions, too, between the exigencies of dealing with diabetes and other demands and desires. In the day-to-day practice of doing bodies such tensions cannot be avoided. Like it or not, they must simply be handled.

The body-we-do is not a whole. Keeping ourselves together is one of the tasks of life. This has implications for what one might ask or expect of medicine. Sullivan has suggested that patients' self-awareness should be added to the results of medicine's own pathological gaze. Our suggestion is different. It is that instead of adding a further layer of knowledge, medicine should shift its self-understanding. Medicine should come to recognize persistently that what it has to offer is not a knowledge of isolated bodies, but a range of diagnostic and therapeutic interventions into lived bodies, and thus into people's daily lives. Even the pathological gaze is not merely a gaze, but involves manipulation. Medicine's activities always concern both what is beneath and what is beyond the skin. But if all medical operations, even if they simply seem to address bodies, are interventions in lives, then they should be appreciated accordingly. Thus not only their effectiveness in improving one or two parameters, but the broad range of their effects deserves self-reflexive attention.[20] Not all of these effects should be expected to be for the better. In articulating how it is doing, in considering the effects of its activities, medicine would be wise to confront its own tragic character: medical interventions hardly ever bring pure improvement, plus a few unfortunate "side-effects"; instead they introduce a shifting set of tensions.

Putting it in this way, we may seem to suggest that medicine's self-reflections should take an ethnographic turn. And so we do.[21] Interestingly, ethnographic methods that foreground practices and draw together disparate entities in a single story aren't new to medicine. In the materials and methods section of research articles practicalities of all kinds (the setting of the intervention in question, the technology mobilized, patient characteristics, and so on) are scrupulously made explicit. It is only in the conclusion that they tend to be forgotten. And listen to the clinical interview: a doctor asks How are you? or What can I do for you? and expects the patient to tell a story about daily-life events in which entities of all kinds (beans, blood, table companions, cars, needles, sugar) coexist and interfere with one another. A good case history, finally, tells about a patient's situation in a language that moves from blood sugar levels to work ambitions to the doses of insulin prescribed to love life to previous operations to saturated fat uptake to temper and if need be back again. Why not tell stories about medicine in a similar way?

Medicine's current self-reflection is predominantly epidemiological in character. Epidemiology brings together disparate entities too, but its method of accounting isolates every so-called variable from all the others and is incapable of articulating links and tensions between them. At this point ethnographic recounting is a more promising technique: it can produce rich stories of lived bodies in which medicine figures as a part of daily life. But smooth narratives that seek to bring coherence will miss the point. If the tragic aspects of living-in-tension and intervening-for-the-best are to be described, jagged story-lines are needed. And they should be told by a variety of narrators whose voices may be drawn together or clash. For this is where patients come in again: aware, not just self-aware, but equally able to tell stories about medicine and the effects of its interventions.[22] The overall aim of a multi-voiced form of investigative story telling need not necessarily be to come to a conclusion. Its strength might very well be in the way it opens questions up.

No, if medicine were to never forget about practicalities again, if it were to attend persistently to the body-we-do, this would not solve all its problems, let alone all problems that plague us, its patients. But even so, it is worth a try.

NOTES

Acknowledgments. Thanks to the people with diabetes and the professionals working with them who were interviewed or observed for this study; and especially, in the Netherlands: to "Miriam T.," Edith ter Braak, Yvonne de la Bije, Willem Erkelens, and Harold de Valk; and in the UK to the staff and patients in an anonymous general practice in the English North West Regional Health Authority area. Thanks to Claar Parlevliet for her interview work, to Alice Stollmeijer for her analyses of food-issues, to Jeannette Pols, Dick Willems, and Ingunn Moser for many discussions on physicalities and subjectivities, and to Bernard Kruithof for comments on an earlier version. This earlier version was also discussed at a Body Theory workshop in Paris and we thank all participants, especially Madeleine Akrich, Marc Berg, and Pascale Brouet and most of all Lise Kvande.

This article is reprinted by permission of Sage Publications Ltd. from *Body & Society* 2004, 10, 2–3: 43–62 (© Sage Publications Ltd, 2004).

1. A variety of classical texts articulated this (now common) knowledge in a variety of different ways; see, for example, Merleau-Ponty (1962) for an analysis which mobilizes the neurology then current to talk about the subject's body image; or Wittgenstein (1953) for the difficulty of talking about pain and other bodily sensations.
2. For a philosophically argued example, see Toombs (1992), and for an example in the mode of social anthropology, see Good (1994). In the literature attention to people's stories about life-events is sometimes given priority over attention to the self-awareness of their bodies. In this text, however, we prefer not to take this way out too quickly, but to respond directly to Sullivan's worry that *the body known by modern medicine is not self-aware.*
3. So in good Foucauldian mode we do not take it that feeling oneself from the inside has always had pretty much its present shape, and was "colonized" or displaced by modern medicine. Rather, the two (subjective and objective knowledge) came into being together. For a wonderful study that allows its readers not simply to understand but also to "feel" how people used to inhabit their bodies differently, see Duden (1991).
4. For this study we gather and analyse a wide range of "materials": medical textbooks; scientific journals; patient journals and information leaflets; advertisements; autobiographical texts. We also ethnographically observe clinics for people with diabetes and interview them and the relevant professionals. In the present paper we focus in particular on the treatment for people with diabetes 1, (early onset diabetes, which always makes people insulin dependent) which is more difficult to "manage" than diabetes 2. Diabetes 1 also tends to come with a higher incidence of hypoglycaemia. The quotes in this article are not supposed to tell the reader about the specificities of the *people* uttering them. Instead they are intended to inform us about *practices*

of dealing with diabetes—practices that are so spread out that they are hard to study ethnographically for a limited number of researchers who have only limited time, and would also prefer not to intrude for long periods into other people's lives by spending days and days with them. So we take professionals as well as people with diabetes as (*lay*) *ethnographers* in their own right, taking it upon ourselves to select, translate, combine, and contrast their stories.

5. Treatment practices for diabetes are by no means universal or even general in the "western world." In a later stage of our study we hope to introduce international comparisons. Since the field work and interviews mobilized in this article are primarily from the Netherlands, we use a Dutch textbook here.

6. However much those working within the phenomenological tradition stress our "being-in-the-world" as bodies, they situate (the understanding of) such bodily being *beside* the representational knowledge *of* bodies; see, for example, Csordas (1994). Building on the tradition of science studies allows us to include representational practices among other practices, each of which is equally mundane. Appreciating the laboratory as a set of practicalities owes most to Latour and Woolgar (1979); its most beautiful explanation and defence is still to be found in Latour (1988). There are, of course, also many studies that unravel the practices of daily life. And some, as we are doing here, move from one site to the other. See the essays in Conein et al. (1993).

7. A possibility which holds most promise for those who have become ill recently: the ability to *feel* a hypoglycaemia coming on may also deteriorate as a consequence of the diabetes.

8. Western medicine depends in many respects on the bodily self-awareness of its patients. In order to allow doctors to use their diagnostic tools properly, patients have to first answer questions such as: what do you feel, where does it hurt, at which moments, is it an itching or a knife-like feeling, and so forth. In all the criticism of medicine's neglect of the patient's *self-awareness* this dependence has been understudied. But see, for example, Strauss et al. (1985) which pays attention to the *articulation work* that patients, like doctors, are engaged in.

9. Eating, in its turn, is linked up with the body in complex ways that obviously go far beyond "countering hypoglycaemia." That studying such mundane sociophysical activities may shed new light on a great many aspects of life is shown in the interesting inquiry into the intertwining of *food* and *memory* by Sutton (2001).

10. For a further exploration of the multiplicity of the objects of medicine that follows from persistently foregrounding practice, with the example of atherosclerosis, see Mol (2002).

11. All knowledge practices depend on the active body knowing, even if a lot of effort has been spent on expelling the relevance of the body from some of them—notably those knowledge practices called "science." For a discussion of this history, and the persistent and variant relevance of knowing-bodies, see the essays in Lawrence and Shapin (1998).

12. As does other knowledge, that of ethnography included. See, for the latter, Stoller (1989).

13. As an extension of this, it would be interesting to analyse medical technology with the theoretical repertoire that has been developed in anthropology for the study of *material culture*. See, for instance Arnoldi et al. (1996).

14. The question of the amount of pain involved in measurement is interesting in its own right. Some of our informants tell that it doesn't hurt *them*. One person remarked that it didn't hurt him because he didn't mind measuring so

much—he said he had the impression that the hurt grows with the aversion. However, if one feels no pain at all, this is not a good sign either: it may indicate that neuropathy has set in and is impairing one's sensitivity.

15. For an experimental investigation into the way difference between self and other is established in people as bodily awareness early in life, see Butterworth (1995).

16. This may, with a slightly different twist, also be called "performing bodies." For a defence of the "performative turn" in the language of philosophy, with the many ways of *doing* differences between the sexes as its target, see Butler (1993).

17. Indeed one of the internists observed and interviewed described a patient of hers who does not want to give up rally diving—a sport that is seriously dangerous for someone with diabetes, because if you get into a hypo it is impossible for others to get you out of it. Somehow living on the edge may, for some people, be too worthwhile to give up. On the combination of risky sports and disabilities, see Moser (2003).

18. In their great attack on the way "Western thought" tries to forget about "the body," Lakoff and Johnson explore many fascinating body-related metaphors, that of "organic wholeness" among them. But while they bring the body *inside* philosophy that has for so long sought to exclude it, it is still as a body we *have* and *are*. Their "body" remains observational, it is not a body we *do*, and it is not metabologic; see Lakoff and Johnson (1999).

19. For a variety of explorations of complexity see the contributions to Law and Mol (2002).

20. This implies that clinical epidemiology is no longer sufficient for the evaluation of medical interventions. For an example that shows how exploring the details of clinical interventions and their various effects may help to not just evaluate but even improve the clinic, see Lettinga and Mol (1999).

21. A self-understanding in which medicine is appreciated as a set of techniques enacting bodies, also helps elsewhere (e.g., to understand the deep divergence between, as well as the possible coexistence of, different medical traditions—such as the "Western" and the "Chinese" tradition); for this see Kuriyama (1999).

22. So far it has mainly been patients who have told stories about their lives with medical interventions together with disease. Other possible participants have been much less forthcoming. One might say that what we argue for here is that the turn to practice that such literature exemplifies, be taken up in professional self-reflection as well (see e.g., Frank 1995; Murphy 1990; and, for an intriguing mixture of daily life stories and a cultural analysis, Stacey 1997).

REFERENCES

Arnoldi, Mary Jo, Christraud Geary, and Kris Hardin, eds. 1996. *African material culture*. Bloomington: Indiana University Press.
Butler, Judith. 1993. *Bodies that matter: On the discursive limits of "sex."* New York: Routledge.
Butterworth, G. 1995. An ecological perspective on the origins of self. In *The body and the self*, edited by José Luis Bermúdez, Anthony Marcel, and Naomi Eilan, 87–106. Cambridge, MA: MIT Press.

Conein, Bernard, Nicolas Dodier, and Laurent Thévenot. 1993. Special Issue on "Les objets dans l'action: De la maison au laboratoire." *Raison Pratique* (Paris) 4.

Csordas, Thomas, ed. 1994. *Embodiment and experience: The existential ground of culture and self.* Cambridge: Cambridge University Press.

Duden, Barbara. 1991. *The woman beneath the skin: A doctor's patients in eighteenth century Germany*, translated by Thomas Dunlop, Cambridge, MA: Harvard University Press.

Foucault, Michel. 1976. *The birth of the clinic: An archaeology of medical perception.* London: Tavistock.

Frank, Arthur. 1995. *The wounded storyteller: Body, illness and ethics.* Chicago: University of Chicago Press.

Golledge, Reginald G. 1997. On reassembling one's life: Overcoming disability in the academic environment. *Environment and Planning D: Society and Space* 15:391–409.

Good, Byron J. 1994. *Medicine, rationality and experience: An anthropological perspective.* Cambridge: Cambridge University Press.

Hirschauer, Stefan. 1993. *Die soziale Konstruktion der Transsexualität: über die Medizin und den Geschlechtswechsel.* Frankfurt am Main: Suhrkamp.

Kuriyama, Shigehisa. 1999. *The expressiveness of the body and the divergence of Greek and Chinese medicine.* New York: Zone Books.

Lakoff, George, and Mark Johnson. 1999. *Philosophy in the flesh: The embodied mind and its challenge to Western thought.* New York: Basic Books.

Latour, Bruno. 1988. *The pasteurization of France.* Cambridge, MA: Harvard University Press.

Latour, Bruno, and Steve Woolgar. 1979. *Laboratory life: The social construction of scientific facts.* Beverly Hills, CA: Sage.

Law, John, and Annemarie Mol, eds. 2002. *Complexities: Social studies of knowledge practices.* Durham, NC: Duke University Press.

Lawrence, Christopher, and Steven Shapin, eds. 1998. *Science incarnate: Historical embodiments of natural knowledge.* Chicago: Chicago University Press.

Lettinga, Ant, and Annemarie Mol. 1999. Clinical specificity and the non-generalities of science: On innovation strategies for neurological physical therapy. *Theoretical Medicine and Bioethics* 20:517–35.

Merleau-Ponty, Maurice. 1962. *Phenomenology of perception*, translated by Colin Smith. London: Routledge & Kegan Paul.

Mol, Annemarie. 1998. Lived reality and the multiplicity of norms: A critical tribute to George Canguilhem. *Economy and Society* 27:274–84.

———. 2002. *The body multiple: Ontology in medical practice.* Durham, NC: Duke University Press.

Moser, Ingunn. 2003. Living after traffic accidents: On the ordering of disabled bodies. Ph.D. diss., University of Oslo.

Murphy, Robert. 1990. *The body silent.* New York: Norton.

Stacey, Jackie. 1997. *Teratologies: A cultural study of cancer.* London: Routledge.

Stoller, Paul. 1989. *The taste of ethnographic things: The senses in anthropology.* Philadelphia: University of Pennsylvania Press.

Strauss, Anselm, Shizuko Fagerhaugh, Barbara Suczek, and Carolyn Wiener. 1985. *Social organization of medical work.* Chicago: University of Chicago Press.

Sullivan, Mark. 1986. In what sense is contemporary medicine dualistic? *Culture, Medicine and Psychiatry* 10:331–50.

Sutton, David. 2001. *Remembrance of repasts: An anthropology of food and memory.* Oxford: Berg.

Toombs, S. Kay. 1992. *The meaning of illness: A phenomenological account of the different perspectives of physician and patient.* Dordrecht: Kluwer.
van Haeften, T. W. 1995. Acute complicaties—hypoglykemische ontregeling. In *Diabetes mellitus*, edited by E. van Ballegooie and R. J. Heine. Utrecht: Bunge.
Willems, Dick. 1998. Inhaling drugs and making worlds: A proliferation of lungs and asthmas. In *Differences in medicine: Unraveling practices, techniques and bodies*, edited by Marc Berg and Annemarie Mol, 105–18. Durham, NC: Duke University Press.
Wittgenstein, Ludwig. 1953. *Philosophical investigations.* Oxford: Blackwell.

6 Sociotechnical anatomy
Technology, space, and body in the MRI unit

Regula Valérie Burri

In recent years, biomedical research and clinical practices have become increasingly dependent on new imaging technologies. The use of digital X-ray, computer tomography, or magnetic resonance imaging (MRI) has changed the ways biomedical knowledge is produced and applied in laboratories and hospitals, and it has transformed how bodies are seen and understood in medicine and society today. These transformations are not only emerging from the employment of images in diagnostic or interventional procedures, or from the adoption and incorporation of visual medical knowledge when patients get to see their body scans. They are also intertwined with the sociotechnical practices by which a medical image is constructed as an artifact within the laboratory or clinical setting. In this article, I focus on the implications of such practices for bodies of patients, technologists, and physicians, which are involved in the process of medical image production. I am interested in how epistemic practices, material conditions, and social norms contribute to the shaping of bodies when an image is fabricated in a specific MRI unit.

Social studies of digital medical imaging have included reflections about the body, while looking at how visual representations are adopted by individuals and incorporated into the knowledge of one's own body (e.g., Duden 1993; Cartwright 1995; Dumit 1997, 2004; Casper 1998; Treichler et al. 1998; van Dijck 2005). Only a few studies, however, have looked at how the body is involved in the very process of medical image production and at how it interacts with machines, instruments, spatial arrangements, social institutions, or other bodies, although laboratory studies and studies in the history of science have pointed to the important role of the body as a tool in the manufacture of scientific knowledge (e.g., Knorr Cetina 1988; Schaffer 1992; Lawrence & Shapin 1998). A physical dimension of medical image production was examined by Amit Prasad (2005), who looked at how the new medical gaze generated by MRI operates in radiologists' laboratories. Kelly Joyce (2005) has shown how the popular narratives used in MRI examinations result in the intertwining of economic interests, physical bodies, machines, and cultural practices in the MRI image. Drawing from ethnographic fieldwork at several MRI units in Switzerland, Germany, and the United States, my essay does not analyze the physicians' discourses and perceptions but rather examines how bodies are constituted in medical imaging by exploring the sociotechnical practices and constellations in which the image production takes place. My multisited ethnography showed that despite the local particularities of the MRI units or contingencies in the clinical organization in different places, some general conclusions can be drawn. The ways the bodies are constituted in the imaging process can be described as an inherent characteristic of the imaging process.

FABRICATING INSTRUMENTAL BODIES

In the process of image production in an MRI unit, bodies are tentatively defined and formed; they are specifically shaped by the local interplay of a set of knowledge practices with machines and social actors. The interaction of epistemic practices and material culture—the distributed agency between actors and technology (cf. Latour 1988, 1993, 1996; Pickering 1993, 1995; Rammert 2003)—shapes the bodies in a specific way in order to make the image production possible. The material objects of the visualization process and the practices of radiologists, technologists, and other physicians are thus disciplining conditions and practices that contribute to the formation and adaptation of the bodies involved in image production, that is, the production of what could be called "instrumental bodies." These bodies are prepared and made instrumental to facilitate the data acquisition necessary for the constitution of a medical image. The fabrication of such "instrumental bodies" is not a reflexive strategy of the social actors, but an intrinsic and contingent moment of the process of image production. It involves the bodies of both patients and medical staff which are, as I show in my essay, somehow refractory to the imaging process and thus have to be adapted to the local sociotechnical setting. Through exploring the material conditions, social norms, spatial arrangements, and professional practices that are parts of the imaging process, my essay analyzes the ways in which such instrumental bodies are constituted in imaging situations.

Based on my observations of the—quite similar—production processes of MRI scans in the different hospitals and research centers I visited, I assume that there is an implicit structure or a modeling principle that is inscribed not only in the techniques, skills, practices, social conventions, and cultural perceptions, but also in the technology, instruments, and other material resources that are part of the visualization process. Drawing on Foucault's notion of "political anatomy" (Foucault 1975/1995), I suggest calling this inscribed structure a "sociotechnical anatomy." In contrast to Foucault's concept, the disciplining effects of this principle are only contingent. The "sociotechnical anatomy" becomes effective in the epistemic practices, the social norms, and the material resources involved in the visual representation of a body in medicine, that is, it inhabits the techniques, practices, and machines deployed in the process of image production. The "sociotechnical anatomy" ensures that the bodies are not only scanned but also simultaneously formed as instrumental bodies during this process. Through analyzing the ways in which instrumental bodies are constituted in imaging situations, I aim to reveal the "sociotechnical anatomy" that is shaping the imaging process. Despite the local particularities of the MRI units or contingencies of the clinical organization in different places, it is the sociotechnical anatomy which engenders the formation, adaptation, and regulation of the body—in other words, its instrumental fabrication.

SPATIAL ARRANGEMENTS

When I entered an MRI room for the first time, the most remarkable thing I registered was the huge size and extravagant design of the machine used in MRI examinations. Imaging apparatuses look like "large metal doughnuts standing up," writes Joseph Dumit, referring to PET scanners (Dumit 2004: 72). The machines occupy a third or even a half of the space in the rooms I visited during my fieldwork. To acquire the necessary data, MRI machines make use of a strong magnet. In order to protect the magnetic field from a disturbing environment that could interfere in the data acquisition process and cause visual artifacts in the images, the scanners have to be put in a separate and well-isolated room. Next to this room—and in contrast to it—a second room is built in every MRI unit from where the scanner and data acquisition are managed. This adjoining anteroom serves as an operations center in which computers, laptops, video monitors, medical equipment, small instruments, and the display portion of an electrocardiogram apparatus are installed next to the console of the scanner. The technologist sits in front of the console and enters a command into the computer. She selects some imaging sequences, such as the number and thickness of the cross-section and the perspective of the images, and customizes them from the console (cf. Burri 2001). Having set these acquisition modalities in the software program, she starts to run the scanner. Simultaneously, she observes the patient on a video screen placed above the console, and from time to time she watches the patient through a window that permits her to see the scanner from the adjoining anteroom. Physicians and technologists are thus able to observe and control the patient during the entire process of acquiring the image data.

In what way does this specific spatial situation of the workplace incorporate what I called the sociotechnical anatomy? From an architectural point of view, the room with the MRI scanner is a separate, isolated place. But it is a room that only makes sense along with another room—the anteroom with the console from where the machine is controlled. As mentioned above, this dependent, hierarchical spatial order can be found in any MRI unit. It implies various dimensions of disciplining coercions and can thus be understood as a materialized form of a disciplining structure, that is, the sociotechnical anatomy. The disciplining aspects of this spatial model can be described as isolation, transparency, invisibility, surveillance, and control. During the data acquisition, the patient is all alone in the room with the scanner. He or she is spatially isolated but is constantly overseen by the technologist. Furthermore, the surveillance is at least twofold: The patient's body can be observed through the window, on the computer screen, and—in the room described above—also from the video display which does not show the mediated transparent body but instead filmed images of the patient lying in the scanner.

This situation reminds the observer of Foucault's well-known description of the Panopticon—the model of a prison designed by Jeremy Bentham at the end of the eighteenth century (Foucault 1975/1995). The Panopticon incorporates a control tower central to an annular building which is divided into cells. The occupants of the cells are isolated from one another and subject to scrutiny by an observer who stays in the tower and remains unseen. The Panopticon thus allows seeing without being seen, which, according to Foucault, ensures the power to work. The spatial arrangement in the MRI unit can be seen as a similar construction. The technologist and the physician are given the power to observe the patient without being seen themselves, and the patient—like the prisoner in Bentham's model—does not know if he or she is actually being watched. Obviously, the consequences are different in the two cases. Unlike the prisoner, the patient is glad to have somebody overseeing and controlling him or her. But in both formations, specific anatomies of disciplining coercions are at work. While in Bentham's design, according to Foucault, the asymmetrical visibility has to be understood as a strategy of exclusion by which governmental power prevails, the architectural model in the MRI unit could be interpreted as a strategy of authority by which the dominance of Western biomedicine is expressed: MRI machines are part of a technoscientific and high-cost health care system that is most widespread in Western cultures; while the United States, Europe, and Japan rely on expensive medical equipment, many societies do not have equal access to such machines.[1]

SEGREGATING MACHINES

In addition to the arrangement of the rooms and equipment, another material structure contributes to the constitution of instrumental bodies while the image is produced—obviously, the scanner is part of this process. In conventional MRI machines, the tube of the apparatus is quite narrow. People who are claustrophobic or disoriented often become fearful or anxious about being confined in such a narrow, body-length MRI tube. As a consequence, in clinical practice it quite often happens that the data acquisition has to be delayed or even stopped because patients become afraid;

around one third of all cited problems that occur during MRI examinations concern the problem of patients who feel anxious or claustrophobic.[2]

It not only takes certain psychological dispositions for patients to be examined in an MRI machine. It also requires of them specific physical properties: a limited size and weight. Not all bodies can be scanned. If they are too tall or big, it might be impossible to fit them into the tube. This, together with the problem of claustrophobia, is the main reason the industry—especially in the United States—has started to increase the production and foster the development of open scanners. The obesity of patients creates problems for imaging examinations. Such bodies might even be refractory to some open systems. In a promotion for a new open scanner, General Electric, one of the leading firms in the production of MRI scanners, quotes the radiologist Jeffrey Rosengarten from Gurnee Radiology Center in Libertyville, Illinois, as follows: "Once we were unable to scan a 450 lb. patient on one of our other open systems, so we sent the patient to our OpenSpeed system and completed the study successfully" (General Electric 2001). Although open systems are improving technically and will be more widespread in the near future, many scanners used today are still closed systems.

Whether a specific body can be examined using MRI depends not only on its size and weight but also on its physical integrity. Bodies which contain metallic implants or pacemakers are usually not allowed to be scanned with MRI, since metallic material often causes image artifacts; in the case of the pacemaker, implanted instruments could be disturbed by magnetic fields and become dangerous for the patient. The use of MRIs as a visualization technology thus implies the adaptation of the bodies prior to the MRI examination. Bodies have to be customized to a specific physical norm, that is, refractory bodies have to be disciplined by forcing them to conform to the image of a "normal," average body which is both physically intact and not too large in weight or size. In other words, the apparatus generates a segregation between bodies that can be scanned and others that cannot. The machine exclusively accepts precursorily disciplined, specifically formed bodies which have already been adapted prior to the MRI examination to what has been socially defined as a norm. The ways in which technical artifacts are produced and designed is shaped by socially negotiated notions, including concepts of normality (Bijker et al. 1987; MacKenzie & Wajcman 1999). This also applies to the construction of medical technology. The building of an MRI machine is dependent not only upon technical possibilities and restrictions but also on engineers' and physicians' perceptions, which have been shaped by what is considered a "normal" body in a specific Western culture. Foucault has shown how such notions of normality and abnormality have shaped knowledge and power relations, and how the definition of "normality" and the processes of "normalization" have extended governmental control over individuals and their bodies (Foucault 1975/1995, 2003). In the case of medical visualization technologies, such concepts are not to be understood as the prevailing power of a nation-state but, again, as an implicit, although powerful, manifestation of Western biomedicine that reinforces existing concepts of normality. The preselection of bodies which can be screened in the MRI room, while other bodies are excluded from such examinations, is part of the entire process of producing instrumental bodies.

COMMUNICATION(S): (RE)ESTABLISHING SOCIAL NORMS

Social norms and local conventions contribute to the disciplining of those bodies which have gained access to the MRI room, bodies that are subjected to specific social expectations. Physicians and technologists expect the patient to be willing to cooperate with the medical staff during the whole imaging process and to comply with all instructions. The patient is expected to remain completely calm during the data acquisition. He or she is not allowed to move in the tube, in order to prevent image artifacts. Thus, the patient must lie still, breathe regularly, not cough, and, if a brain scan is taken, not even move his or her eyes. He or she is also expected to follow the instructions of the technologist, who stays in the control room during the entire examination. The expectations regarding the behavior of the patient are communicated in various ways; it is possible to distinguish between explicit and implicit communications. Explicit communications include written instructions and verbally communicated directives. Most hospitals or clinics provide written information about the MRI apparatus and the respective examination on their websites. The patient is thus not only given the details of the technique and the procedure but also told how he or she should behave. "The Patient Guide to the MRI Scan," for example, a brochure made available online by the Massachusetts General Hospital (MGH; n.d.), gives several instructions:

> You should arrive 15 minutes before your scheduled appointment. This allows time for you to complete any necessary paperwork, change your clothes for your scan and answer questions from our technologist about your medical history before we start your scan.... (7)

> If you are wearing anything metallic, such as jewelry, dentures, glasses, or hearing aids, that might interfere with the MRI scan, we will ask you to remove them. You should not have your credit cards in your pockets during the scan because the MRI magnet can affect the magnetic strip on the card. Patients who are having a brain scan should not wear make-up as some brands contain metal.... (8)

It is important for you to lie very still and, at some points, you may be asked to briefly hold your breath as the picture is taken. (MGH n.d.: 9)

Such directives are also listed on an information sheet that is provided by most MRI units. The sheet is delivered once the patient arrives at the unit or, in some places, during an earlier consultation between the doctor and the patient. Just like the website guide, the information sheet also tells the patient how to behave in the tube. In most countries, the sheet has to be signed prior to the examination since informed consent is required to perform the imaging. Explicit communications also include oral instructions. At Massachusetts General Hospital, a representative of the MRI Department calls the patient the day before the examination to provide all the information needed. Often, the patient has a conversation with his or her doctor prior to the examination, during which the doctor explains how the imaging procedure is accomplished. This talk also includes briefings concerning what the patient is expected to do. Finally, during the imaging process the technologist, who is connected to the MRI room by an intercom system and a microphone, constantly instructs the patient what to do; for example, when to hold his or her breath during data acquisition.

In addition to these explicit and formalized communications, social expectations and conventions are also conveyed by implicit communications. In the MRI units I observed, the radiologist entered the MRI room shortly before the data acquisition was started. The patient was already lying on the table and prepared for the examination. When the physician said hello and asked the patient how he or she and the family were doing, this was more than just him trying to be nice. By means of this small conversation, the physician intended to calm the patient, who often felt a bit anxious or at least tense; even more importantly, the conversation served as a marker to signal that the situation was now entering a new stage, that is, that the explicitly communicated expectations would now apply. By this implicit communication of social norms, the explicit norms were thus reinforced. At the same time, social expectations and norms which had never been explicitly formulated were also transferred—such as the expectation that the patient should remain in the tube during data acquisition. Although this expectation seems too evident to require an explicit instruction, it quite often happens in clinical practice that patients try to leave the tube or to free themselves from the equipment.[3]

In fact, both explicit and implicit communications address the patient in a way that imposes self-discipline. The patient is expected to have his or her body under control and to overcome any anxiousness he or she might have when lying in the tube. This form of body control—the self-disciplining of the body—is another practice contributing to the production of the body in its instrumental form. By the explicit and implicit communication of expectations, social norms are (re)established and contribute to the fabrication of instrumental bodies.

SOCIOTECHNICAL CONSTELLATIONS

A great deal of technology is involved in the production of images. It is not only the MRI machine that is needed; other medical tools and instruments, like a machine to check breathing or an instrument to measure blood pressure, are also required in order to perform a tomography. Furthermore, the MRI scanner itself consists of many different components.

The interconnection of body and technology

To begin data acquisition, the patient has to be positioned on a patient table that is controlled by a computer. He or she is then connected to the various apparatuses. The sensors for measuring blood pressure and for taking the electrocardiogram have to be applied to the body. A special belt to check breathing is put on the patient. Often some special components of the scanner—so-called surface coils—have to be placed on the body as well. This interconnection of body and technology can even be invasive: In many cases, a contrast agent is administered to the patient intravenously, and the syringe is placed on the table behind the patient's head. This injection helps to enhance the visualization of certain regions of the body, and it is required when an angiogram of the vessels is produced. Once the patient is connected to the various apparatuses and instruments, his or her body is covered with a blanket. Occasionally, the patient is also offered head-phones in order not to be forced to hear the loud knocking noises of the machine. Since the surface coils and the breathing belt are constricting and the injection brings the patient's arm in a fixed position, the freedom of action of the body is restricted. The patient's body is now fixed, stabilized, and made immobile—that is, it is disciplined and made instrumental in order to begin data acquisition.

The Spatial Stabilization of Bodies

Using Foucault's (1975/1995) framework, such an interconnection of body and technology could be understood as a connection between a body and a manipulated object in which the relation between the body and the object is defined by what Foucault calls a discipline, that is, a specific set of techniques to discipline and control social bodies. In contrast to Foucault's example of objects such as weapons, the objects in the medical imaging process, for example the MRI scanner or the surface coils, are not manipulated by the patient but are controlled by a radiologist or a technologist in the adjoining room. From this sociotechnical constellation and from the social position of the actors involved in the imaging process, a specific spatial distribution of the bodies emerges: The patient stays in the MRI room, the technologist sits in front of the console in the control room, and the physician is often in constant movement—he walks around, leaves the adjoining room for a couple of minutes to visit the ward, returns, talks to the technologist, and then walks over to work at another computer. This distribution of bodies is due not only to the technical conditions but also to the social and professional positions of the actors involved in the production of an image. During data acquisition, the configuration of bodies is temporarily stabilized. The patient stays in the tube, and the technologist does not usually leave the console while the data is being acquired. This configuration is established in a habitual and practical sense and is not reflexively produced; it is part of an implicit, routinized, and incorporated imaging practice, that is, it is the outcome of implicit knowledge (cf. Polanyi 1958, 1967) and of what Bourdieu (1980/1992, 1972/2002) calls a practical sense.

The spatial configuration and stabilization of the bodies can be seen as another disciplining practice that emerges from the sociotechnical anatomy. It creates a sociotechnical constellation that defines a specific spatial relation among the bodies of the involved actors and between these bodies and the technology. It is not only the body of the patient that is tentatively fixed and disciplined; the sociotechnical constellation also stabilizes the bodies of the technologists and physicians, which are also constructed as instrumental bodies that work toward the production of a medical image.

WORK ROUTINES: STRUCTURING THE IMAGING PROCEDURE

In addition to the spatial constellations, the practices that structure the imaging procedure and its time flow also contribute to the fabrication of instrumental bodies. These practices are part of a professional and habitual work routine. This refers, for example, to the way in which the patient is brought into the scan room and prepared for the examination, and to the epistemic practices involved in the procedures of data acquisition.

Being geared to standards and efficiency

Performing these practices, radiologists and technicians are oriented to professional standards and criteria of efficiency. Among the most prominent examples are the locally produced standard protocols, which define what specific type of image has to be produced for a specific indication. This is necessary because the acquisition modalities for the images have to be selected in the software program: for example, the number and thickness of the cross-sectional images or the perspective and resolution of an image. The standard protocols define how such modalities are usually handled; for example, how many sequences of data acquisition should be taken if the proposed diagnosis is, say, ischemic heart disease. The protocols are made and are regularly adapted and revised by radiologists and physicians working with MRI at a local unit. Stefan Timmermans and Marc Berg (1997, 2003) have pointed to the importance of standards in medicine and have shown how medical protocols may permit a "local universality" to be achieved. In the MRI units I observed, the protocols consisted of a number of computer printouts stapled together. The technologists only checked this "book" once in a while, when a more unusual data sequence had to be taken. The most important directives, however, had become part of their daily work routine and had thus been incorporated by them as integral parts of their implicit knowledge.

Standard protocols enhance the efficiency of the whole imaging process. Without protocols, physicians would have to give detailed instructions for each image, and this would take them a long time. Time efficiency was considered a very important criterion in every MRI unit I visited. A work schedule is used to indicate which patient is to be screened at what hour of the day. In larger MRI centers, this schedule cannot be always followed, since emergency patients drop in and outpatients cancel their appointments. Nevertheless, the schedule ensures that technologists do not have to waste time and are able to proceed efficiently. Both the use of standards and the desire for efficiency structure the sequence and time flow of the imaging process. Both orientations thereby involve the adjustment of the patient's body to a given routine practice. This adjustment is part of the body's instrumental characteristic.

Remote commands

Finally, the imaging procedure is structured by the technologist's remote commands during data acquisition. Using the intercom system with the microphone that connects the control room to the MRI room, the technologist constantly tells the patient what to do. Before starting the sequence, the technologist asks the patient if everything is okay and informs him or her that the procedure is beginning. The technologist observes the curve of breath on the monitor in front of her. She gives her instructions according to the trajectory of this curve: "Now please breathe in...breathe out...breathe in...breathe out...and now please hold on...." The patient stops breathing, the curve on the monitor declines, and the technologist starts the sequence. Through such instructions, the process of data acquisition is structured, and the activities of the patient's body are controlled. Periodically, the technologist comments on the cooperative behavior of the patient. After fifteen seconds of held breath, the technologist turns on the microphone again and says, "Okay, now please go on breathing. You are doing very well!" Such acclamations are repeated whenever the acquisition of a sequence is finished. These words, which serve to encourage the patient lying in the tube, can also be understood as an acknowledgment of the patient's compliant and cooperative behavior; they serve to constantly qualify the self-disciplining of the patient and thus enforce the instrumental production of his or her body.

CONCLUSION

In this article, I have analyzed the implications of the production of a medical image for the bodies involved in this process. I have argued that the practices, social conventions, and material resources which are involved in image production imply the creation of a temporary disciplined, "instrumental body." I have assumed that despite local particularities, there is an implicit structure or modeling principle that is inscribed not only in the techniques, social norms, cultural perceptions, and material conditions but also in the technology, instruments, and design of the setting that are involved in the visualization process. This inscribed and modeling principle—the "sociotechnical anatomy"—has a teleological character. Its implicit purpose is to discipline the body, that is, produce an instrumental body, in order to adjust it and adapt it to a sociotechnical system that serves a specific interest: the accumulation of biomedical knowledge about the body. In this sense, the sociotechnical anatomy could be interpreted as a manifestation of the power of scientific biomedicine, consisting of an increasingly visio-technoscientific access to the body that defines the ways bodies are seen and understood in Western cultures.

NOTES

Acknowledgments. The chapter is based on the paper "Digitalizing, Disciplining: Imaging Practices and the Constitution of the Body in Biomedicine," which was presented at the annual meeting of the Society for the Social Studies of Science, Milwaukee, WI, November 8, 2002. I thank Joe Dumit for his comments and Kim Hays for editing the manuscript.

1. OECD Health Data show that huge differences also exist among Western countries. While the United States had a total of 13 CT and 8 MRI scanners per million people at their disposal, Japan had 94 CT and 35 MRI scanners per million (in 2001 and 2002, respectively). However, countries like Turkey and Hungary (in 2002, 8 CT and 3 MRI per million and 7 CT and 3 MRI per million, respectively) do not have the same infrastructural access (OECD 2004; numbers rounded).
2. In a study among medical institutions in Switzerland working with MRI, around one third of all cited problems that occurred during MR examinations referred to patients who felt anxious or claustrophobic (Burri 2000).

3. Around 8 percent of all problems that occur during MR examinations concern patients trying to leave the tube or to free themselves from the equipment (see Burri 2000: 77). This behavior is, in most cases, due to anxiety or
claustrophobia caused by the machine's narrow tube and the knocking noises
heard during data acquisition.

REFERENCES

Bijker, Wiebe, Thomas Hughes, and Trevor Pinch, eds. 1987. *The social construction of technological systems: New directions in the sociology and history of
technology.* Cambridge, MA: MIT Press.
Bourdieu, Pierre. 1972/2002. *Outline of a theory of practice*, Cambridge Studies
in Social Anthropology, no. 16. Cambridge: Cambridge University Press.
———. 1980/1992. *The logic of practice.* Stanford, CA: Stanford University Press.
Burri, Regula Valérie. 2000. *MRI in der Schweiz: Soziotechnische, institutionelle
und medizinische Aspekte der Technikdiffusion eines bildgebenden Ver-
fahrens*, Preprints zur Kulturgeschichte der Technik, no. 10. Zürich: ETH.
———. 2001. Doing images: Zur soziotechnischen Fabrikation visueller Erkenntnis
in der Medizin. In *Mit dem Auge denken. Strategien der Sichtbarmachung in
wissenschaftlichen und virtuellen Welten*, edited by Bettina Heintz and Joerg
Huber, 277–303. Zürich: Springer, Edition Voldemeer.
Cartwright, Lisa. 1995. *Screening the body: Tracing medicine's visual culture.*
Minneapolis: University of Minneapolis Press.
Casper, Monica J. 1998. The *making of the unborn patient: A social anatomy of
fetal surgery.* New Brunswick, NJ: Rutgers University Press.
Duden, Barbara. 1993. *Disembodying women: Perspectives on pregnancy and the
unborn.* Cambridge, MA: Harvard University Press.
Dumit, Joseph. 1997. A digital image of the category of the person: PET scan-
ning and objective self-fashioning. In *Cyborgs and citadels: Anthropologi-
cal interventions in emerging sciences and technologies*, edited by Gary Lee
Downey and Joseph Dumit, 83–102. Santa Fe, NM: SAR Press.
———. 2004. *Picturing personhood: Brain scans and biomedical identity.* Princeton, NJ: Princeton University Press.
Foucault, Michel. 1975/1995. *Discipline and punish: The birth of the prison.* New
York: Vintage Books.
———. 2003. *Abnormal: Lectures at the College de France, 1974–1975*, edited by
Mauro Bertani and Alessandro Fontana. New York: Picador.
General Electric. 2001. GE Reaches Milestone with 75th OpenSpeed MRI Magnet, Company News, News Releases, September 28, 2001. http://www.
gemedicalsystems.com/company/pressroom/releases/pr_release_4985.html
(accessed November 23, 2005)
Joyce, Kelly. 2005. Appealing images: Magnetic resonance imaging and the production of authoritative knowledge. *Social Studies of Science 35*, no. 3: 437–62.
Knorr Cetina, Karin. 1988. Das naturwissenschaftliche Labor als Ort der "Ver-
dichtung" von Gesellschaft. *Zeitschrift für Soziologie 17*, no. 2: 85–101.
Latour, Bruno. 1988. Mixing humans and nonhumans together: The sociology of
a door-closer. *Social Problems 35*, no. 3: 298–310.
———. 1993. *We have never been modern.* Cambridge, MA: Harvard University
Press.
———. 1996. *Der Berliner Schlüssel. Erkundungen eines Liebhabers der Wissen-
schaften.* Berlin: Akademie Verlag.

Lawrence, Christopher, and Steven Shapin, eds. 1998. *Science incarnate: Historical embodiments of natural knowledge.* Chicago: University of Chicago Press.

MacKenzie, Donald, and Judy Wajcman, eds. 1999. *The social shaping of technology,* 2nd ed. Buckingham, UK: Open University Press.

Massachusetts General Hospital, Imaging Services. n.d. The patient guide to the MRI scan. http://www.mghmri.org (accessed March 12, 2006).

OECD. 2004. OECD Health Data 2004, cited by ECHI (European Community Health Indicators) project. http://europa.eu.int/comm/health/ph_information/dissemination/echi/echi_en.htm (accessed August 12, 2005)

Pickering, Andrew. 1993. The mangle of practice: Agency and emergence in the sociology of science. *American Journal of Sociology* 99, no. 3: 559–89.

———. 1995. *The mangle of practice: Time, agency, and science.* Chicago: University of Chicago Press.

Polanyi, Michael. 1958. *Personal knowledge. Towards a post-critical philosophy.* Chicago: University of Chicago Press.

———. 1967. *The tacit dimension.* Garden City, NY: Doubleday Anchor.

Prasad, Amit. 2005. Making images/making bodies: Visibilizing and disciplining through magnetic resonance imaging (MRI). *Science, Technology, and Human Values* 30, no. 2: 291–316.

Rammert, Werner. 2003. Technik in Aktion: Verteiltes Handeln in soziotechnischen Konstellationen. In *Autonome Maschinen,* edited by Th. Christaller and J. Wehner, 289–315. Wiesbaden: Westdeutscher Verlag.

Schaffer, Simon. 1992. Self-evidence. *Critical Inquiry,* 18, no. 2: 327–62.

Timmermans, Stefan, and Marc Berg. 1997. Standardization in action: Achieving local universality through medical protocols. *Social Studies of Science* 27, no. 2: 273–305.

———. 2003. *The gold standard: The challenge of evidence-based medicine and standardization in health care.* Philadelphia: Temple University Press.

Treichler, Paula A., Lisa Cartwright, and Constance Penley, eds. 1998. *The visible woman: Imaging technologies, gender, and science.* New York: New York University Press.

van Dijck, José. 2005. *The transparent body: A cultural analysis of medical imaging.* Seattle: University of Washington Press.

7 Risk and safety in the operating theater

An ethnographic study of sociotechnical practices

Cornelius Schubert

The sociological study of sociotechnical systems is most often linked to risks, failures, accidents, or catastrophes, be they in concrete systems failure such as in nuclear power plants, air and sea traffic (Perrow 1987), space flight (Pinch 1991), or the more abstract relations of society and technology (Beck 1986; Luhmann 1991). Sociological analysis usually starts when something has gone wrong or danger seems imminent. In this essay, I would like to address the issue from a different angle. It is not a question of analyzing which factors have contributed to an accident or of finding somebody who caused it, but rather of studying the activities which were undertaken to avoid danger and compensate failure.

Hutchins has done this in the case of navigation systems failure on board a U.S. Navy ship (Hutchins 1996). He argues that in case of failure, the tasks and relations of components in a sociotechnical system are reconfigured to compensate for the failed subsystem. In the following sections, I will analyze yet another sociotechnical system, namely, the surgical operating theater (OT). The study is based on ethnographic observations and video recordings and interviews in large and small hospitals in Germany and Australia. It is partly based on an interdisciplinary discussion between sociologists, semioticians, psychologists of work and organization, and computer scientists with the aim of analyzing and modeling safety-relevant cooperation in complex sociotechnical systems.[1]

SAFETY AND COOPERATION IN THE OPERATING THEATER

Drawing on research conducted in so-called workplace studies (cf. Knoblauch & Heath 1999), I will focus mainly on describing and analyzing the practices and activities displayed in the local situation of the OT, especially in the field of anesthesia (cf. Pettinari 1988; Fox 1994). Patient safety is regarded as a product of medical teamwork. It is a result of complex inter-relations between humans and machines and is deeply rooted in the local practices of doctors and nurses. Thus, this analysis relies to a large extent on in situ observation.

Classical safety engineering proposes to gain safety through standardization: a preformed solution for already known or anticipated problems. This approach is dominant in industrial production, but is also prominent in medicine, where guidelines, protocols, and good medical practice serve to maintain a high standard of health care. On the other hand, the work of doctors and nurses is inevitably subject to variability and change when they have to adapt actions, for example a treatment, to an individual patient. The interplay of stability and flexibility is therefore a key characteristic of cooperation in medical settings.

Many medical sociologists have commented on the incomparability of workflows in industrial plants and hospitals (Rohde 1974; Siegrist 1978) with reference to the low potential for standardization of individual work and for cooperation in hospitals. The term *cooperation* has mainly been used in the sociology of work, dating back to Marx (1968). Marx used the term to describe how the (industrial) work of many is conduced according to a systematic (production) plan. Later, cooperation was also understood to be determined by machines and technology in many ways (cf. Popitz et al. 1957).

Cooperation is conceptualized as a prearranged order of mutually dependent subtasks; its function is to integrate the diverse elements of industrial work created by the division of labor. As with standardization and safety, this is only partly true for medical practice. Work in hospitals is only partly determined by external rationales; this observation led Strauss to coin the term *negotiated order* (Strauss et al. 1963) in order to stress the importance of specific, local interactions in structuring work.

The approaches of Marx and Strauss pretty much represent two counterpart positions when it comes to studying the role of technology in work settings. Technological determinism highlights the power technology has over people, whereas social constructivism elaborates the formative force of social affairs (for a discussion on medical technology, see Timmermans & Berg 2003). The following sections will neither stress the first nor the second approach, but aim to combine empirical data and analytic concepts for a better understanding of work in high-tech settings. Cooperation in operating theaters inevitably depends on the use of machines and instruments. That is why I will examine the interrelations of humans and machines more closely in my analysis. The main question to be answered is how the workflow in a cooperation is organized.

DIFFERENT MODES OF COOPERATION

In this section, safety issues such as order, structure, flexibility, and adaptation are central. Safety-relevant activities in the OT are most often a collective effort of small teams: In anesthesia, the team usually consists of an anesthetist, an assisting nurse, and some technical appliances.

My analysis is concerned with the questions of how system disturbances are dealt with before they develop into irreversible accidents, how problems are dealt with, and how order is restored. Fortunately, serious accidents are very rare in the observed hospitals. However, the daily work of OT personnel seems to be riddled with small disruptions of the workflow. These minor disturbances are so frequent that they are considered as being part of the routine by most team members. Nonetheless, the analysis of everyday work can reveal many interesting aspects about the structure of teamwork and the interactivities with machines.[2] That is why I will concentrate my observations on the planned, scheduled, and common operations.

I propose to distinguish three modes of cooperation under the aspect of safety: routine, compensation, and improvisation. These modes are categories of observable activities. They also serve as analytic terms to typify different states in the management of disturbances in the workflow. They are based on a pragmatic view of human action (cf. Dewey 1922), and are developed to describe interindividual events rather than intrapersonal processes. Therefore, the emphasis is on observable mechanisms of cooperation.

Routine

Most problems of everyday work are dealt with by applying routines (cf. Berg 1992: 169; Strauss 1993: 191). In the OT, routines also take up the lion's share of activities. The routine activities that will be discussed now are those used to coordinate standard steps of work.

Routine work consists of standardized patterns of activities employed on a regular daily basis. Cooperative tasks like intubations, handling patients, and interacting with anesthetic machines are usually deeply embedded in everyday work routines. This is how the team sustains and fulfills consistent mutual expectations of how work should be done with very little coordinative effort. These standardized patterns of activity are the result of the legal framework and medical guidelines on the one hand, and are produced by local interactions and interactivities over time on the other hand.

Research in other areas, such as control rooms (Heath & Luff 1992), shows that the situational routines and problem-solving practices of personnel are likely to predominate over the official standards that are written down in manuals. The routines not only are confined to the relations between humans, but also emerge out of the interactivity with machines. Experienced anesthetists often have their own way of using certain machines, turning off pesky alarms, or bypassing annoying safety features. This does not mean that patient safety is diminished or neglected. The anesthetists are reducing the amount of information and possible sources of distraction in order to be able to concentrate on what is relevant to them.

Alarms are usually visible as well as audible, so turning off the sound will not turn off the alarm entirely.

This also means that the team and the technology are mutually tuned to one another. It is a process of reciprocal alignment.[3] Once the participants work as a good team and their pattern of activities is aligned, cooperation is swift and effective. Furthermore, these sociotechnical routines prove to be quite durable and resistant to change. The trade-off between flexibility and structure plays a significant role in patient safety: The advantages and disadvantages of both need to be balanced in order to guarantee safe procedures.

In the social sciences, the observation of routine activities under the aspect of safety is underdeveloped in comparison to the study of breakdowns and accidents. Patterns of routine coordination can be briefly described in the following way: There is almost no or very little verbal exchange about the task between the members of the team. The interactivities with machines are well trained and happen silently and quickly.[4]

People generally use gestures to indicate their expectations to one another. A quick glance or a short movement of the hand is sufficient to organize the cooperation. An impressive example of nonverbal coordination is the interaction between two surgeons when stitching. One surgeon usually assists the other, and if they both have enough experience, the assisting surgeon will coordinate his actions merely by looking at his colleague's hands. The same goes for experienced nurses, who are able to judge doctors by their actions and engage in cooperation with them by themselves. In such cases, the organization of cooperation relies on a high degree of overlapping knowledge (cf. Hutchins 1996: 265); that is, anesthetists, surgeons, and nurses share a certain amount of knowledge concerning the others' tasks. Their actions are thus mutually accountable, and the coordination is swift.

To sum up, routines as problem-solving patterns form a major part of everyday work. They represent successful and well-established solutions of frequent problems, and serve to sustain consistent expectations within the team. They grow out of interactions and situations, and once in practice they are likely to remain a resource for further actions. When observing routine cooperation, the communicative aspects of coordination are mainly contained in gestures and facial expressions. There is little task-related verbal exchange, and actions intertwine at a relatively high speed.

Compensation

But what happens when routines fail to deliver the desired result? In most cases, there are backup strategies. I call this kind of coordination "compensation." Backup strategies are, like routines, patterns of action preformed to fit a specific situation.

Compensation strategies can be acquired by training or experience. In many cases, the personnel are trained to respond to a specific problem in an appropriate manner. Based on emergency plans, for instance, anesthetists train to cope with uncommon but possible situations like ventricular fibrillation. These emergency plans are constructed like algorithms. Their precise and sequential instructions serve to guarantee quick and correct reactions in time-critical situations. Compensation can then be described as using a set of alternative routines. They differ from the daily patterns of action in the aspect that they are not internalized by practice, but by additional exercise.

In addition to the trained algorithms, there are local forms of compensation that stem from experience. The practice of rebooting is, for example, one strategy that has been proven successful in daily work in order to deal with malfunctions of microelectronic devices. Also, malfunctioning perfusors are switched off and on, again in the hope that the problem will disappear. This practice does not come from manuals or guidelines, but is the product of ongoing interactions with computers. Solving the breakdown of a technical system is mainly a process of countervailing failed machine processes with compensatory human action. The first step is to substitute the dysfunctional component, and then the component's original functionality needs to be restored. This can be done in two ways: either by trying to repair the component or by exchanging it for another one. In the OT, both strategies are used according to the failed component's size: Small components are exchanged, and larger components are repaired.

Coordinating compensatory action is thus a matter of signaling a change of strategy to team members. The routine problem-solving pattern is replaced by a different pattern. Compensation can be regarded as a failsafe or backup mechanism, designed to counteract expected problems.

In the phase of compensation, the team displays a particular behavior. If technological failure is involved, activities are usually repeated: Unsuccessful routines are reiterated several times, until a change of strategy is considered. This repetition is a sign for commencing problems and, if noticed, will serve as a signal for other team members to adapt their patterns of action. Hesitation is another signal, displaying uncertainty about how to continue. Both activities, repetition and hesitation, do not draw the attention of others directly toward the problem. They are subtle markers of a disturbance in the workflow and are only picked up if a person pays attention to what another person is doing. In the OT, nurses who notice such a small disturbance are likely to interrupt their own work and get ready to assist the doctor. Being ready to intervene, they let the situation develop to see whether their help is needed.

Thinking aloud is a little less subtle behavior, but it serves well to direct the attention of others toward a problem without having to ask explicitly for help. Anesthetists who think aloud make their actions or problems noticeable to the nurse or uninvolved team members.

The above examples highlight the subtle nuances of coordination during the phase of compensation. The distinction between routine and compensation is an analytical one. In real-life situations, routine and compensation merge into one another. Compensation is considered to be part of the daily grind by most staff members and not a deviance from usual business. Compensation is a source of local variations in working practices, because many strategies and patterns of actions have evolved out of situational contexts and are specific to local culture.

Improvisation

As I have mentioned earlier, routine and compensation are preformed solutions to certain problems. In addition to expected problems, unanticipated disturbances might occur. In such a case, the team must develop a new solution on the spot. In contrast to standard problem-solving strategies, this is called "improvisation." This term stresses the importance of the situational resources and real-time changes during cooperation (cf. Becker 2000 for some critical thoughts on the order of improvisation).

Since unexpected problems are encountered on the basis of available means, improvisation is tied to specific situational constraints; for example, machines, tools, media, and personnel. During an improvisation phase, the relations of components are reconfigured according to the breakdown. The reconfiguration is a reorganization of cooperation and requires particular forms of coordination. Since there are no commonly shared preformed strategies, the explicit exchange of verbal communication is central to this mode of cooperation. Improvisation often relies on direct verbal orders to adapt patterns of action to suit the situation. Order is restored step by step in a negotiated process through the interactions of components as a potential solution that unfolds out of the situation (cf. Hutchins 1996: 317). Of course, if the team is very experienced, improvisation can also happen on a nonverbal basis by gestures and glances. In the case of technical systems failure, it is necessary to establish a quick substitute for a defective component, especially if the patient's life depends on it; for example, in the case of artificial ventilation. OT technology is usually designed to be redundant, and many machine functions can be replaced by human action if the components are loosely coupled (cf. Perrow 1987). When observing improvisation, one can see that actions are discontinued and problems are being verbalized. Also, there are questions and queries concerning the breakdown. It is in this stage of uncertainty that reconfiguration occurs. The contingencies of the situation need to be reduced until work can be resumed.

In the context of structure and flexibility, the situational reconfiguration of patterns of action is central to understanding work practices in complex settings. The maintenance of a stable phase turns out to be a key feature of everyday work since it is also quite significant for the patient's safety. The maintenance of a stable phase can be considered as a form of repair work, as work that is performed in addition to anesthesia and surgery in order to maintain a safe course of action.[5]

Strauss et al. added sentimental work as an aspect of patient care (Strauss et al. 1982) and error work in respect of counteracting the development or the consequences of mistakes (Strauss et al. 1985: 242). In the light of the present study, repair work should be considered a related aspect of work, especially if medical technology is involved. Since the process of coordination and reconfiguration involves machines as well as humans, their activities are closely interrelated and interwoven. In the next section, I will look at these relations in more detail.

SOCIOTECHNICAL ENSEMBLES

As argued above, the classical concepts of cooperation, work, and division of labor have their shortcomings once the presumption of technological determinism is dropped. The order of cooperation changes according to the situation and is dependent on local activities. To be able to make abstractions from this observation, some analytical aspects have to be taken into account. In this respect, the elements of the ensemble on which the reconfiguration is based deserve closer attention.

Following the approaches of technology in action (cf. Rammert & Schulz-Schaeffer 2002; Rammert 2003) and likewise technology in practice (Timmermans & Berg 2003), the operating theater is conceptualized as a sociotechnical ensemble. I use "ensemble" here instead of "system" to avoid confusion with large-scale concepts dealing with nuclear power or air traffic as such. Sociotechnical ensembles are hybrid networks in the sense that they enclose human as well as technological components and that relations between the components are significant to its specific function (cf. Bijker 1995: 269). Also, the term *ensemble* is used to characterize the real-time coordinative tasks undertaken by the individual members, very much like the performance of a musical or theatrical ensemble. The OT can thus be conceptualized as one hybrid network among many within the organization of a hospital.

Narrowing the argument further, sociotechnical ensembles refer to a situation located distinctly in time and space. The ensemble's components are real individuals and objects. Their specific characteristics, particularities, skills, knowledge, and functions are the elements constituting the ensemble.

Going into more detail concerning the reconfiguration and the operating mode of the ensemble, I will now emphasize the interweaving of activities during cooperation. Some research has been conducted on the tacit order of teamwork (Hindmarsh & Pilnick 2002), analyzing how anesthetists organize their actions in the presence of a conscious patient. The following observations indicate that this kind of order is kept up even after the patient is under anesthesia. I will examine the role of technological objects in both interaction and interactivity and will as well analyze the tacit order. My main concern will be to examine how ensembles establish reliable procedures in spite of the high variability of their actions, and how knowledge is distributed within the ensemble.

A rather unexpected observation made in the OT was the high level of deviation from the classic division of labor of doctors and nurses. Using subtle ways and techniques, nurses have a larger part in the organization of teamwork than is officially granted to them. For instance, a young nurse might ask a chief doctor to lift a patient's legs so she can prepare the operating table. Masking an order as a question does not destroy official hierarchy, and the doctor can help without losing face (cf. Goffman 1999). A surgeon might ask a nurse which instruments he should use, or an anesthetist might ask a nurse for her opinion on how to administer narcotics. Nurses tend to be in the OT most of the time and acquire knowledge concerning surgery, anesthesia, and the general organization of work. Sometimes, it is the nurses who rearrange patients' schedules according to organizational requirements, anticipating surgeons' needs and considering past, present, and future events. As a collective, nurses acquire, store, and relay relevant information on patients, operations, machines, and so on.

In particular situations, experienced nurses might know more than novice doctors. Looking at cooperation in such situations, it is interesting to see whether and how nurses can pass on such knowledge without corrupting the traditional doctor–nurse relationship.

In many interviews, anesthetists have had a story to tell about an old nurse they met when they were beginners. This nurse was either an indispensable source of helpful information or, in unfortunate cases, a strong force better not to be messed with. Either way, nurses play an important role in anesthetists' early careers. In analyzing the work practices in operational theaters, it is important to look at the relations between nurses and doctors that have effects on the work outcomes; that is, patient safety.

When working with experienced anesthetists, nurses are likely to show respect. They do this by waiting for the anesthetist to give them an order—also often masked as a question—before they act. When working with novice anesthetists, though, nurses often take a more active part in cooperation.

A video recording of an intubation performed by a novice anesthetist and an experienced nurse revealed the subtle reconfigurations of the ensemble. The intubation is a procedure where a plastic tube is inserted into the patient's throat, so that artificial respiration can be conducted. Usually, the nurse has the role of an assistant, but here she is informally in charge of the intubation, leading the young doctor through the process, preparing instruments, and anticipating and avoiding possible difficulties. She seems to be one step ahead of the doctor and, by supplying him with the right instruments at the right time, indirectly structures the cooperative workflow.

In one incident of the video recording, the nurse holds onto the plastic tube, even after handing it over to the doctor. The doctor is puzzled at first, but the nurse keeps holding onto the tube. By holding onto the tube, she is trying to get the anesthetist's attention on the shape and position of the tube in his hand, then she lets go. The activity of handing over the tube therefore takes as much as four seconds. Thus, she does not just hand over the tube, but also hands it over in the correct shape and position for the doctor to insert it into the trachea. The doctor is "taught" without being "told." Positioning the tube is an interactive task involving the doctor, the nurse, and the tube. In this particular incident, the reconfiguration of the ensemble is necessary, because there is an asymmetry in knowledge between the doctor and the nurse. The nurse knows which shape the tube has to have to be inserted correctly, because she is experienced and well trained. For his part, the doctor has to accept the nurse's help and play along. The tube turns out to be more than just a medical instrument: It is a medium through which knowledge is transferred.

Similar processes can be observed in microsurgery. Surgeons often do not tell novices how to hold the camera; instead they grab their hands, manipulate them, and tell the assistants they want to have it "like this." Certain forms of practical knowledge are difficult to be put into words, so teachers do without them. Knowledge is directly passed on in a configuration of bodies and tools.

The above examples show that cooperation in sociotechnical ensembles is influenced by three factors: (1) the actual activities of personnel; (2) their interindividual experience; and (3) personal know-how.

Cooperation can be understood as a process in which data, information, and knowledge are produced, shared, transformed, stored, and passed on. Thus, the relation of knowledge to cooperation has a considerable effect on the reconfiguration of sociotechnical ensembles.

1. The maintenance of a stable phase is only possible through the active adaptation of activity patterns. As I have observed, nurses possess substantial knowledge about working in the OT, and adaptation to disturbances is faster and more reliable the more knowledge is mutually shared. The classic concept of the division of labor does not account for these variations in competence, and the subtle ways of bypassing hierarchies are only observable in the real situation. We can see how legal constraints and organizational needs function as the background for actual cooperation. They are invoked in critical situations, for example under stressful circumstances or when chains of command are useful for synchronizing actions, but they only have a limited effect on everyday work.

Just as human action differs from the formal norms, the use of technology also varies from the engineers' intentions. Technology is used in local contexts and on the basis of common beliefs and practices. Stories are told about unreliable machines, and young doctors are confronted with episodes where technological failure has led to tragic events. In one hospital, for instance, staff members in the waking room like to work without extensive technology. They rely on their medical skills and use only pulse oximetry and blood pressure cuffs to gather machine-mediated data on the patient's vital functions. In an interview, the acting chief of staff told me that they had made a collective decision to reduce medical technology in favor of their clinical skills. I was also told that in comparison to waking rooms with more technology, they performed just as well in terms of patient health. The maintenance of a stable phase is no doubt partly dependent on the OT's social order, but as we see, it also relies on the way in which machines are tied into the network of human action. Stability comes from technical or social routines and in most cases from both. Since the balance between the two has no optimal state, there is no one best way of achieving and sustaining patient safety. Technology can be replaced by humans, and vice versa. Culture and individual beliefs are key factors in organizing cooperation and determining the shape and function of hybrid networks. Today, technological dominance is apparent in most large Western hospitals, and the study of evolving hybrid networks will gain in importance as this trend increases: Balancing the advantages and weaknesses of these networks is of great importance to patient safety.

Distributed knowledge as a constitutive element of these ensembles is contained not only in rules, guidelines, and records, but also in the stories, anecdotes, and episodes passed on from one doctor or nurse to the next. The narrative structure of medical knowledge has been analyzed by only a few researchers (cf. Atkinson 1995; Hunter 1991) and certainly deserves closer attention.

2. Cooperation is also based on interindividual experience. Staff members interact on the basis of a common history and use their knowledge about the skills and abilities of other team members to organize cooperation. Their history contains past interactions and the results of these interactions evolving over time. History helps to establish trust, or sometimes distrust, between team members. It generally makes their actions mutually accountable and leads to safe and effective cooperation, and thus to the formation of routines.

Interindividual experience also enables the emergence of overlapping knowledge. The process of overlapping often occurs in a reversed order of hierarchies, that is, people with less status acquire knowledge usually associated with higher status. Such a learning process is fundamentally situated in local culture. Only if doctors share their knowledge and extend the rights and duties of nurses can this distribution of knowledge take place. Knowledge then becomes attached to experience rather than status, and the more experienced the team members are, the safer the work becomes.

History and overlapping knowledge also shape teams' social structures. They establish practices and provide collective routines for tackling everyday problems, and prove to be highly resistant to change. Once relations within the team are made durable by interindividual experience so that members know what to expect from each other, their relations are unlikely to change, but are reinforced during following interactions.

Sociotechnical ensembles display a tendency to standardize actions and interactions. Previous successful actions serve as blueprints for future actions. Undoubtedly, these elements constitute what can be called good team cooperation, but on the other hand they can lead to undesirable consequences, for example what social psychologists have called groupthink and risky shift—the tendency to adopt a simplistic, cohesive view of a situation or to make more dangerous decisions. Again, a balance is needed between a well-tuned team and the ability to make changes if necessary.

3. Personal know-how is the other important aspect of cooperation comprising one individual's experience. Experts define situations differently in comparison to novices. An anesthetist summed up the relationship between knowledge, experience, and action in an interview: "You have to know a lot to do nothing." This seems to be a paradox, but it describes the conjunction between knowledge and action very well. Experience changes the experts' perspective on events. The boundary between what is acceptable and what is not becomes less solid and more dependent on other observations, that is, data are triangulated and interpreted before action is taken. Personal know-how establishes idiosyncratic frames of relevance that soften formal regulations. In a situation where a patient might seem critical to a novice, an experienced anesthetist can still be in control; for example when sudden changes in treatment might actually harm the patient or symptoms are due to the side effects of medication and will be of short duration.

Expert knowledge is largely implicit (Polanyi 1983) and is more like a sure instinct or rule of thumb. That makes it different from the explicit knowledge that novices acquire during formal education and training. Research on expert systems has shown that it is not easy to transform implicit expert knowledge into explicit guidelines and rules (Rammert et al. 1998). Experience, however, makes experts resistant to novel definitions of situations (Wagner 1995). They tend to stay in their tracks instead of trying to integrate new or inconsistent information.

Once expert knowledge is transformed into guidelines or microelectronic devices, it is easily accessible by novices, giving them an advantage by bypassing years of learning. A novice sufficiently equipped with technology can deliver the same level of quality care as an expert who might not need or want all these gadgets and devices.

As I have stated above, experts use technology based on their experience. Anesthetists might turn off alarms that they consider irritating or useless, considering the patient as the primary source of information and technology only to be a subsidiary one. As long as the patient has red lips (enough oxygen), small pupils (enough narcotic medication), and a dry, warm forehead (no stress), he or she is well.

Machines transform vague impressions and inferences about a patients' state into discrete numbers and graphs. Anesthetic monitoring provides accuracy at the price of introducing a possible source of error; for example, a sensor falling off, a tube becoming blocked, or a program error occurring. Experienced anesthetists therefore do not take monitoring at face value, but judge it on the perceived credibility of the source (cf. Cicourel 1990). They try to integrate data into a larger framework based on other observations, experience, and personal know-how. Thus, anesthetic monitoring is used and valued according to individual experience and operative requisites. During a short and simple operation, one does not need heavy monitoring equipment, but it is indispensable during long and complex procedures. Novices tend to focus more on the technical equipment than on the patient, whereas trained experts, especially in large hospitals, try to balance direct and mediated monitoring. In an interview, when asked if there is a difference between novices and experts, an anesthetist put it like this: "Of course, that is completely clear. First, everyone only looks at the monitor, like being magnetized. That happens automatically, I did the same in the beginning. And after that comes experience."

Over time, anesthetists develop individual practices of how to use and judge technological artifacts. This is especially notable if, for instance, old and experienced doctors perform routine anesthesia. In some cases, they will turn down most of the alarms and perform artificial respiration by hand, because they feel closer to the patient this way. They express the view that monitoring technology, in a way, blocks their perception of the condition of the patient. These experienced old-fellows were trained without a great deal of technological equipment and very much like to rely on their own five senses.

The maintenance of a stable phase, interindividual experience, and personal know-how reveals the subtle, local, and individual elements and constraints of interaction and interactivity in sociotechnical ensembles. Interaction is based on the perceived credibility and ability of the other. Cooperation changes as the ensemble's components change. The components, humans as well as machines, are embedded in the context of local culture. Their actions and activities are tightly interwoven with one another. They form a hybrid network, whose ties are set up and configured in action by staff and machines. Knowledge is distributed across the team and various media and machines as a key element of cooperation. Experts' implicit knowledge is often passed on in stories and anecdotes or in nonverbal fashion. Knowledge can be embodied in technology, gestures, looks, or bodily configurations; it is knowledge in action, constantly being produced, transferred, stored, retrieved, and changed within the ensemble.

CONCLUSION

The above observations and arguments are an attempt to conceptualize activities in high-tech work situations, with a special focus on safety and cooperation issues. The perspectives of cooperation in action and the balancing of stability and flexibility provide an analytical and thematic framework for understanding interaction and interactivity in sociotechnical ensembles. The balance between stability and flexibility is one of the foremost safety issues concerning cooperation in the OT; the team's performance in situ as observational category and analytical perspective emphasizes the flexible character of everyday work.

The term *repair work* should be considered as a wildcard or variable, needing further study and definition. The main point of this is that the focus of work is shifting within sociotechnical systems of medicine away from the well-documented doctor–patient relationship toward the hybrid networks and sociotechnical ensembles of doctors, nurses, patients, and technologies. In analyzing specific sociotechnical ensembles, repair work and the maintenance of a stable phase turn out to be significant elements in cooperation and factors relevant to patient safety.

Further research is indicated in the areas of safety practices, distributed knowledge, and the embedding of technological objects in social contexts. The latter has been described in workplace studies to some extent, though the analytical and theoretical implications have been less explored.

One interesting topic could be the transformation of the profession of anesthesiology through medical technology. This has been done for other fields of medicine looking at different technologies; for example, ultrasound (Yoxen 1989), the stethoscope (Lachmund 1992), or MRI (Burri 2001). Following the concept of the clinical gaze (Foucault 1996), anesthetic monitoring technology enables the doctors to see where they used to be blind. Where the darkness could only be poked at by interpretation and inference, it is now pierced by the precise and objective numbers and graphs of monitoring technology. The use of these technologies in operating theaters and intensive care units and their impact on anesthetic work remain relatively unexplored.

Another set of practices that should be studied more carefully are teams' safety practices. How do members organize safe procedures, and what are their perspectives on safety? Heath et al. have pointed out how awareness is configured in centers of coordination (Heath et al. 2002). In the OT, awareness is also a key element of patient safety: Changes in the patient's state need to be noticed and, if necessary, relayed to the relevant person. Surgeons, anesthetists, and nurses comment on the patient's state, make hints, or verbalize their observations in order to make somebody else aware. These practices are dependent on the workplace situation, and safety practices in the OT might differ significantly from those in intensive care units or other wards. Preliminary observations indicate the existence of different safety regimes, that is, the organization of safety practices in local contexts. An anesthetist described the differences between patient care in the OT and the intensive care unit as being comparable to the difference between driving a sports car and navigating a cargo ship. In the first case, reactions are quick and direct, whereas in the latter one, effects of actions are delayed in time and have multiple contributory factors.

The distribution of knowledge could also be a subject for further research, especially in the training of novices in teaching hospitals. There seems to be a gap between the clear, explicit knowledge taught in universities and the somewhat messy and ambiguous practice of medicine, a phenomenon that can be observed in many if not all fields of applied science (cf. Delamont & Atkinson 2001). How novices are socialized into their future fields of activity and how they go from being novices to becoming experts are topics worth examining. In this context, the relevance of stories, anecdotes, and episodes should be considered in more detail.

The importance of local practices for patient safety has become obvious. Empirical findings can be used to propose a novel way for formally describing cooperation in high-tech work settings, a way in which the emphasis for organizing cooperation lies on situational adaptation rather than prearranged structures and processes. Considering safety as a product of sociotechnical ensembles helps to build a dynamic understanding of situations. Furthermore, an analysis of how hybrid networks of cooperation function is indispensable in understanding how they might fail. A detailed analysis can inform future safety engineering in designing safer and more robust and error-tolerant systems. Local practices and deviations from the norm should not be seen as a threat to but as a resource for safety.

This is where the challenge lies in modeling such systems. An abstract description of coordination and cooperation needs to include all the variations in the workflow and all the contingencies and uncertainties of the local situation to be able to deliver an accurate account of the sociotechnical ensemble. The research done so far is a first step and will continue, because it is becoming more and more important with the increasing participation of machines in patient diagnosis and treatment.

NOTES

Acknowledgments. I would like to thank all staff and patients for their cooperation and patience, as well as the administrations of the hospitals for allowing me to conduct the research.

1. This perspective was developed in the RISK project (Routines and Risks of Distributed Action), which was part of the larger interdisciplinary project KOSIS (Cooperation and Safety in Sociotechnical Systems) at the University of Technology in Berlin.
2. In order to describe the complex interrelations between humans and machines, I will use a classification proposed by Werner Rammert (1998), reserving the term *interaction* for the relationship between humans and the term *interactivity* in respect to the relation of humans and machines.
3. Mead has stressed the importance of interaction in *games* to develop a functional self for the individual (Mead 1975: 107). In teams there are similar processes of socialization that bind the members and help to establish the alter egos as meaningful partners of interaction. In analogy, interactivities with physical objects, like devices and media, establish a sociotechnical order where persons learn to take the perspective of machines like perfusors in order to establish a hybrid network of cooperation (Rammert 1998).
4. I have discussed the methodological implications of this elsewhere (Schubert 2002).

5. The term *repair work* has previously been used by Jörg Potthast to describe the work of maintenance personnel in an international airport and their collective identity in respect to technology (Potthast 2001).

REFERENCES

Atkinson, Paul. 1995. *Medical talk and medical work: The liturgy of the clinic.* London: Sage.

Beck, Ulrich. 1986. *Risikogesellschaft.* Frankfurt am Main: Suhrkamp.

Becker, Howard S. 2000. The etiquette of improvisation. *Mind, Culture, and Activity* 7, no. 3: 171–76.

Berg, Marc. 1992. The construction of medical disposals: Medical sociology and medical problem solving in clinical practice. *Sociology of Health and Illness* 14, no. 2: 151–80.

Bijker, Wiebe E. 1995. *Of bicycles, bakelites, and bulbs: Toward a theory of socio-technical change.* Cambridge, MA: MIT Press.

Burri, Regula Valérie. 2001. Doing images: Zur soziotechnischen Fabrikation visueller Erkenntnis in der Medizin. In *Mit dem Auge denken. Strategien der Sichtbarmachung in wissenschaftlichen und virtuellen Welten*, edited by Bettina Heintz and Joerg Huber, 277–303. Zürich: Springer, Edition Voldemeer.

Cicourel, Aaron V. 1990. The integration of distributed knowledge in collaborative medical diagnosis. In *Intellectual teamwork: Social and technological foundations of cooperative work*, edited by Jolene R. Galegher et al., 221–42. Hillsdale, NJ: Lawrence Erlbaum.

Delamont, Sara, and Paul Atkinson. 2001. Doctoring uncertainty: Mastering craft knowledge. *Social Studies of Science* 31, no. 1: 87–107.

Dewey, John. 1922. *Human nature and conduct.* New York: Modern Library.

Foucault, Michel. 1996. *Die Geburt der Klinik. Eine Archäologie des ärztlichen Blicks.* Frankfurt am Main: Fischer.

Fox, Nicolas J. 1994. Anaesthetists, the discourse on patient fitness and the organisation of surgery. *Sociology of Health and Illness* 16, no. 1: 1–18.

Goffman, Erving. 1999. *Interaktionsrituale.* Frankfurt am Main: Suhrkamp.

Heath, Christian, and Paul Luff. 1992. Collaboration and control: Crisis management and multimedia technology in London underground line control rooms. *Journal of Computer Supported Cooperative Work* 1, no. 1: 24–48.

Heath, Christian, et al. 2002. Configuring awareness. *Computer Supported Cooperative Work* 11: 317–47.

Hindmarsh, Jon, and Alison Pilnick. 2002. The tacit order of teamwork: Collaboration and embodied conduct in anesthesia. *The Sociological Quarterly* 43, no. 2: 139–64.

Hunter, Kathryn Montgomery. 1991. *Doctors' stories: The narrative structure of medical knowledge.* Princeton, NJ: Princeton University Press.

Hutchins, Edwin. 1996. *Cognition in the wild.* Cambridge, MA: MIT Press.

Knoblauch, Hubert, and Christian Heath. 1999. Technologie, Interaktion und Organisation: Die Workplace Studies. *Schweizerische Zeitung für Soziologie* 25, no. 2: 163–81.

Lachmund, Jens. 1992. Die Erfindung des ärztlichen Gehörs. Zur historischen Soziologie der stethoskopischen Untersuchung. *Zeitschrift für Soziologie* 21, no. 4: 235–51.

Luhmann, Niklas. 1991. *Soziologie des Risikos.* Berlin: de Gruyter.

Marx, Karl. 1968. Kooperation. MEW Band 23: *Das Kapital*, vol. 1, 341–55. Berlin: Dietz Verlag.

Mead, George Herbert. 1975. Sinn/Spiel, Wettkampf und der (das) verallgemei-
    nerte Andere. In G. H. Mead, *Geist, Identität und Gesellschaft*, 107–22,
    187–206. Frankfurt am Main: Suhrkamp.
Perrow, Charles. 1987. *Normale Katastrophen. Die unvermeidbaren Risiken der
    Großtechnik*. Frankfurt am Main: Campus.
Pettinari, Catherine Johnson. 1988. *Task, talk, and text in the operating room: A
    study in medical discourse*. Norwood, NJ: Ablex.
Pinch, Trevor J. 1991. How do we treat technical uncertainty in systems failure?
    The case of the space shuttle Challenger. In *Social responses to large techni-
    cal systems*, edited by Todd R. La Porte, 143–58. Dordrecht: Kluwer.
Polanyi, Michael. 1983. *The tacit dimension*. Gloucester, UK: Smith.
Popitz, Heinrich, et al. 1957. *Technik und Industriearbeit. Soziologische Untersu-
    chungen in der Hüttenindustrie*. Tübingen: J.C.B. Mohr.
Potthast, Jörg. 2001. Kollektive Identität und Technik. Die Wartungstechniker
    von Roissy. In *Kollektive Identitäten und kulturelle Innovationen*, edited by
    Werner Rammert, 197–217. Leipzig: Universitätsverlag.
Rammert, Werner. 1998. Giddens und die Gesellschaft der Heinzelmännchen. Zur
    Soziologie technischer Agenten und Systeme Verteilter Künstlicher Intelli-
    genz. In *Sozionik. Soziologische Ansichten über künstliche Sozialität*, edited
    by Thomas Malsch, 91–128. Berlin: Sigma.
———. 2003. *Technik in Aktion: Verteiltes Handeln in soziotechnischen Konstel-
    lationen. TUTS WP-2-2003*. Berlin: Technische Universität Berlin, Institut
    für Soziologie, Techniksoziologie.
——— et al., eds. 1998. *Wissensmaschinen. Soziale Konstruktion eines technischen
    Mediums. Das Beispiel Expertensysteme*. Frankfurt am Main: Campus.
———, Schulz-Schaeffer, Ingo. 2002. Technik und Handeln. Wenn soziales Han-
    deln sich auf menschliches Verhalten und technische Abläufe verteilt. In
    Können Maschinen handeln? edited by Werner Rammert and Ingo Schulz-
    Schaeffer, 11–64. Frankfurt am Main: Campus.
Rohde, Johann Jürgen. 1974. *Soziologie des Krankenhauses. Zur Einführung in
    die Soziologie der Medizin*. Stuttgart: Ferdinant Enke Verlag.
Schubert, Cornelius. 2002. *Making interaction and interactivity visible: On the
    practical and analytical uses of audiovisual recordings in high-tech and
    high-risk work situations. TUTS WP-5-2002*. Berlin: Technische Universität
    Berlin, Institut für Soziologie, Technology Studies.
Siegrist, Johannes. 1978. *Arbeit und Interaktion im Krankenhaus. Vergleichende
    medizinsoziologische Untersuchungen in Akutkrankenhäusern*. Stuttgart:
    Ferdinand Enke Verlag.
Strauss, Anselm. 1993. *Continual permutations of action*. New York: de Gruyter.
——— et al. 1963. The hospital and its negotiated order. In *The hospital in modern
    society*, edited by Eliot Freidson. New York: Free Press.
——— et al. 1982. Sentimental work in the technologized hospital. *Sociology of
    Health and Illness* 4, no. 3: 254–78.
——— et al. 1985. *Social organization of medical work*. Chicago: University of
    Chicago Press.
Timmermans, Stefan, and Berg, Marc. 2003. The practice of medical technology.
    Sociology of Health and Illness 25, no. 3: 97–114.
Wagner, Gerald. 1995. Die Modernisierung der modernen Medizin. Die "episte-
    miologische Krise" der Intensivmedizin als ein Beispiel reflexiver Verwissen-
    schaftlichung. *Soziale Welt* 46, no. 3: 266–81.
Yoxen, Edward. 1989. Seeing with sound: A study of the development of medi-
    cal images. In *The Social Construction of Technological Systems*, edited by
    Wiebe E. Bijker, 281–303. Cambridge, MA: MIT Press.

Part III
Biomedical knowledge in context

8 Genomic susceptibility as an emergent form of life?

Genetic testing, identity, and the remit of medicine

Nikolas Rose

Do we today inhabit an "emergent form of life"? The term *form of life* was made most famous in the work of Ludwig Wittgenstein, but my use of it is hardly a rigorous application of Wittgenstein's argument. By a "form of life," I simply mean to point to the rules and premises for "behaving ourselves," for conducting a life; that is to say, the ways in which our forms of conduct are linked to ways in which we understand ourselves and others; to our sense of what we can hope for or what we must fear; to our ways of judging right and wrong, desirable and undesirable; and also to our conceptions of our obligations toward others and toward ourselves. I also like the term forms of life because it links this reference to the ways in which one may conduct one's life, to another sense—that implied by the idea of a "life form." That is to say, it relates to the question of what we are today, as creatures, as life forms or living beings. In this essay, I want to suggest that there are some intriguing new links between our forms of life and our sense of ourselves as particular life forms.

In identifying such links, I do not mean to imply that there is a simple causal connection between, say, new biomedical or genetic concepts and new ways of living. This is why I use the term *emergence*. The idea of emergence has become popular with the increasing interest in "complexity theory," but once more I use the term rather loosely, simply to refer to something new, which arises not from a single event or discovery, but often unexpectedly and contingently at the intersection of multiple pathways. I like the term *emergence* because it stresses that there are no necessary relations between the different pathways which happen to coincide at a specific point. Something new arises when a series of often quite distinct developments intersect, interact, crash into one another, combine, and redivide, and so on. Sometimes, not always, something novel takes shape as a result. That is the kind of image that I am trying to convey in this term emergent forms of life.

Where are these emergent forms of life taking shape? In relation to biology, and in particular in relation to biomedical biotechnology, which is the central topic of this essay, I suggest one of the pathways involved concerns the changing circuits of biovalue and the shifting relation of biovalue to biopolitics. I borrow the term *biovalue* from Catherine Waldby (2000), who uses it to describe the ways in which a surplus of value can be derived from the vital capacities of living organisms. Carlos Novas and I (2000, 2004) have suggested that the suffix value, here, needs to be understood as encompassing not just economic value but also values of many other sorts, including, of course, the value of health itself to an individual, a family, and indeed a nation. Novas and I also argued that, today, the creation of biovalue should be understood within a shift in the production of biological knowledge and related biotechnologies—a shift in which the "public value" that shaped their production for many decades has been displaced by other measures and criteria of value. Over the last few years, key areas of knowledge, production, and technological development in the field of biotechnology have moved, at least in part, from public science and the work of charitable foundations to private science, mobilized, at least in part, by the search for profits. Simultaneously, politicians, policy makers, think tanks, and others now frequently make the argument that biotechnology is, or should be, a "key national, economical priority." It is identified as such not only in the advanced industrial countries of the West, but also in the countries emerging from the breakup of the Soviet Union and indeed in rapidly developing nations such as India and China. In all these areas, one sees new alliances forming between state, market, and science, as politicians, both national and local, come to believe that in some way or another, the future prosperity of their countries, their region, or their city depends upon its occupying a leading place within the new market for biotech. And, hence, developing biopolitical rationalities embody a new obligation for politicians—their obligation to encourage both public and private investment in bioscience, biomedicine, and biotechnology. These developments are also being embodied in the new sets of relations that are emerging between universities, and scientific researchers based in those universities, and privately funded corporations.

In all these new and intriguing relations, health, the quest for health, the quest for the values that can be produced by health, has become one of the key determinants for biomedical truth. If one has a path-dependant theory of truth, as I do, then it becomes clear that that some of the basic truths articulated in the biomedical sciences are being shaped, in part at least, by research and development directed by the search for biovalue, by beliefs and expectations about the potential for the extraction of value—economic, moral, professional, political—from the very vital character of human life itself. In the process, we are seeing the reshaping of needs, of demands, and of markets for biomedicine, with the hope that new domains, perhaps even an unlimited field, will open for the operation of biomedical biotechnology. That is to say, a field that is not limited by the question of illness and cure but extends much more widely to the management of the very vitality of human existence, that is to say, to life itself. And of course in this new field of needs, demands, and market, a key role is played by the reshaping of biomedical expectations held by individuals, families, and groups, not only in the West but also in developing countries, as consumers of health care and medicine, as consumers demanding cures and having a say in the very nature and direction of medical research itself.

Novas and I framed this in terms of a shift from public value to biovalue, to suggest that the agendas of the bioscientists and biomedicine are not shaped solely, or even mainly, by the priorities and aspirations of public bodies, whether these are publicly funded research councils or government agencies. They are being configured in a new field in which public values and economic values are inextricably intertwined. In order to understand this emergent form of life, therefore, we have to move beyond analyses in terms of bioethics to questions of biopolitics, bioeconomics, and what Paul Rabinow (1992, 1996) has termed "biosocialities."

TECHNOLOGIES OF LIFE

Many have noted that contemporary technologies of life are not simply concerned with normalization or cure, but also make possible the manipulation and transformation of the vital processes of human existence themselves. These have been the focus of much popular scientific and bioethical speculation. I would like to consider these developments more soberly, and to trace them along two axes—those of susceptibility and those of enhancement. What is meant by referring to developments here as "technologies of life"? These involve technologies in the narrow sense, that is to say, equipment and technique. But they also involve technologies in a wider sense, what I would call "human technologies." By a human technology, I mean an assembly of knowledges, instruments, artifacts, persons, practices, and spaces, structured by a practical rationality, which is governed by a more or less conscious goal and underpinned by specific presuppositions about human beings, what they are, and what they could be. Contemporary technologies of life embody futurity. They try to bring potential vital futures into the present and seek to make them amenable to calculation, and then amenable to transformation in the present in the name of an enhanced future. And they are future oriented in another sense. That is to say, they shape and they thrive on a promissory culture of hopes and expectations—a culture in which hopes and expectations of many parties, of individuals, of their families, of governments, of scientists and researchers, of health care organizations and insurers. Of course, there are also the hopes and expectations of biomedical and biotechnology companies for major advances that will not just increase market share but also increase the market itself.

BEYOND GENETIC DETERMINISM

One key mutation in this emergent form of life is a shift in genetic reasoning itself, a shift embodied in the shift in terminology from genetics to genomics and postgenomics. As is well-known, critics of genetics have long argued that simple genetic determinism was a naïve form of reductionism. They asserted, I think quite correctly, that the search for explanations in terms of single genes and their alleles or mutations ignored the complex developmental, social, and environmental processes by which phenotypes were generated. They pointed out, again correctly, that in relation to disease, single-gene disorders were a minority, and that genetic determinism could not account for the emergence and epidemiology of common complex disorders such as ischemic heart disease, stroke, or diabetes. And they argued, again correctly, that simple genetic determinism was even less able to account for conditions whose very definitions and borders were in dispute—such as intelligence, schizophrenia, or depression. Hence, the critics asked why there was such a focus on genetic research; they approached all those who sought to engage in such research with what one might term a "hermeneutics of suspicion." However, if we are considering questions of genetics today, it is very important to recognize a fundamental shift that has occurred in the epistemology and the ontology of genetics.

As we know, heredity was central to the forms of political life from the mid-nineteenth century to the mid-twentieth century. Arguments about heredity were initially framed in terms of the inheritance of character or constitution, and did not make a very clear distinction between inherited and acquired characteristics, often suggesting that physical or moral harm done during one's life as a consequence of illness, debauchery, or vicious conduct could be passed down to future generations, as in the initial formulation of theories of degeneracy. With the rise of eugenics, there was a clearer insistence that it was a biological inheritance that determined human characteristics, both physical and moral. And, as we know, the units of this biological inheritance came to be designated "genes." Hence Evelyn Fox Keller has aptly named the twentieth century "the century of the gene" (Fox Keller 2000). That is to say, it was the century in which a particular entity, first hypothetical and then located on the chromosomes, was seen as both the unit of inheritance and the unit of developments. A gene, in one of a small number of allelic states, would both pass down a character from one generation to another and would govern the development of that characteristic in the individual who possessed that particular version of the gene. As we know, this kind of argument found its apotheosis in the "gene for" paradigm, with the suggestion that there was one "gene" for every characteristic of every living organism. These arguments gained a new prominence from the 1960s to the end of the twentieth century with the more general rise of informational styles of thought and an infatuation with computers and computer programs. This generated a new metaphorical language for genetics: genes were understood as "digital instructions" for making human beings, and hence it appeared that to "decode the genome" was to "read the book of life."

At this time, most geneticists believed that there were between 100,000 and 140,000 human genes, an estimate that made it at least plausible to consider that there might be one gene for each significant characteristic. Other significant elements of this style of thought were the arguments that each disease might be in some way linked to a single, genetic mutation and, similarly, that each protein was coded for by one gene. And finally, of course, there was the central argument that there was no path back from the cell to the gene—the determination was one way only. This is what led some, like Walter Gilbert, to believe that the Human Genome Project embodied a "vision of the grail"—it held the secrets of human existence. However, developments in genomic science proved that this vision—whether fantasy or nightmare—was an illusion. As the work of sequencing the genome reached its fruition, it became clear that the human genome had too few coding sequences for there to be one for each characteristic, or each illness—instead of the 100,000 to 140,000 human coding sequences that had been predicted, when the public Human Genome Project and Celera Genomics simultaneously published their sequences in 2001, each estimated the figure as close to 30,000; more recently, in 2004, that estimate was reduced to between 20,000 and 25,000. The implications were illustrated in a report in *Nature* highlighting the publication of the paper by the human genome sequencing consortium entitled "Finishing the Euchromatic Sequence of the Human Genome." This news item, entitled "Humans Have Fewer Genes," remarked upon the fact that while humans have only 20,000 to 25,000 genes, a fruit fly, using the same form of reckoning, has 13,600; the famous "worm" *C. elegans* has 19,500; rice has 45,000; and maize has 50,000 coding sequences identified as genes. The implication was clear: there is no relationship between the complexity of an organism and the number of coding sequences on its genomes.

In examining human differences, the focus moved from the gene to single nucleotide polymorphisms or SNPs, that is to say locations in the sequence where there was a single substitution of a base, say, a "G" for a "T," or an "A" for a "C," and where this substitution might have functional significance. While the human genome is estimated to contain 3 billion base pairs, and there are only 0.1 percent differences between any two randomly selected individuals, genomic scientists suggest that this amounts to perhaps 15 million differences at the SNP level. Thus one key focus of research is on these differences at the SNP level, differences that are hypothesized to affect both disease susceptibility and drug response. Other complexities soon entered the picture: alternative splicing, epistasis, epigenesis, genomic plasticity, the role of noncoding RNA and much more. It was now clear that one protein could arise from the interactions of sequences on several genes, that one coding sequence could be involved in the synthesis of several proteins, that coding sequences could be expressed in different ways in different cells and at different points in the development and life history of the organism and much more. The focus of postgenomics extended from genes and SNPs themselves to the processes whereby transcription took place (transcriptomics) and to the process of protein synthesis (proteomics). In other words, the attention moved from "the gene" to the cell and the organ, and to complex developmental processes that occurred over time. Further, given the ways in which gene expression is modulated, it became clear that there were indeed many paths from the cell back to the DNA. The language of genes still has a function in the styles of thought of postgenomics, but the close of the twentieth century was indeed the end of the century of "the gene."

What are the social implications of this shift? One of the most significant is the move from genetic determinism to genomic susceptibility. One can already identify a number of "vectors," which are spreading the theme of genomic susceptibility into various practices. One vector is reproductive medicine with the increasing use of genetic testing in advice to prospective parents, in preimplantation genetic diagnosis and elsewhere. A second vector is the potential use of presymptomatic genetic screening for susceptibilities to diseases such as breast cancer. Many have raised concerns about the implications of such screening for issues of informed consent, confidentiality between relatives, and the potential consequences of such predictive information on disease susceptibility in relation to employment and insurance. As yet there is little evidence of the widespread use of such presymptomatic screening except where there is existing evidence of inherited diseases in a family. Nor is there much reliable evidence of such information playing a part in decisions by employers or insurers, although surveys in some countries suggest that this prospect is generating anxiety among actual or potential patients. However, we are already seeing calls for presymptomatic screening of children for vulnerability to psychiatric conditions, coupled with proposals for preventive intervention before symptoms arise. A third vector for the spread of the idea of susceptibility is pharmacogenomics—the search for genetic markers that will predict response to drugs or the likelihood of adverse reactions. Many clinical trials of new drugs already include a pharmacogenomic element, in which genetic analysis is used to try to identify those in the study who respond well or badly, and hence to allow the correlation of genomic information with drug response. The hope here, of course, is not only to be able to "target" drugs more precisely to different population groups, but also to develop diagnostic tests to be used in clinical settings to determine which of a number of potential drugs should be prescribed for a particular individual. Some still speak of fate as "written in the genes" and potentially decipherable by genetic tests. But variations at the SNP level rarely generate determinism and certainty. They indicate probabilities and uncertainties—assigning a given individual to a group that has, say, an 80% chance of responding well to a drug, or a

29% chance of having no response. It is this age of uncertainty that we are now entering.

It is very likely that many biomedical practices will seek to make use of the kinds of "premonitory" knowledges generated by genomic testing. Premonitory knowledges, as Margaret Lock has termed them, are knowledges that seek to bring potential vital futures into the vital present and make them calculable (Lock, 2005). Such knowledges of the future, even an uncertain and probabilistic future, generate obligations—obligations to act in the present upon oneself, one's body, and one's health in relation to those potential futures. To the extent that genomic medicine begins to identify SNP-level variations that increase susceptibility to common complex disorders—rather than simply focusing on diseases with a major genetic component—this will have implications for the forms of life led by the many and not the few, for all of us have some susceptibilities which are or might be in the future potentially knowable. Thus, all of us are potentially candidates for the form of life of the susceptible self.

What form might this form of life take? It would be a form of life where the responsible citizen would have the obligation to know and manage his or her life of susceptibilities—a kind of permanent management of genomic uncertainties. It would entail a new and ongoing relation with medical authorities, not just at times of frank illness, but before illness manifested itself, or perhaps when illness would never manifest itself, but nonetheless in relation to the uncertain premonitions generated by these new kinds of knowledge. In these circumstances, one would imagine an expansion of the pastoral role of medical and paramedical authorities, a role in which they would seek to advise and guide individuals in the proper ways of living with those uncertainties and managing their vital lives in relation to a potential but uncertain vital future. In such a form of life, the powers of doctors and the apparatus of medicine would extend out from the domain of illness and cure to the management of life itself.

Some critics, commenting on the rise of genetic testing for future diseases, have suggested that this will usher in an age of "enlightened impotence" and a new kind of fatalism; that is to say knowledge of the future without the power to alter it. However, evidence from the United States and from Europe suggests that quite the reverse is taking shape. Far from involving impotence and fatalism, genomic information is becoming the grounds for action and for intervention. In this new field of molecular medicine and genomic information, biology is not destiny but opportunity. Many of those who are undertaking research and development, especially commercial development, in relation to genomic medicine dream of a future of personalized, predictive, and preventive medicine. But the reality is not a world of certainty, but of uncertainty, a world of risks, a world of probabilities, and a world in which new definitions of risk groups, of risky families, and of at-risk individuals might take shape. The forms of life being developed here are those that Carlos Novas and I have described in terms of "biological citizenship," that is to say of individuals and groups claiming their rights and struggling in the micro politics of health and in the macro politics of health care systems for funding, for research, and for provision in relation to their own particular conditions (Rose & Novas 2000, 2004). This is a citizenship that also confers obligations: The biological citizen is one who not only demands something from others, but also must exercise a certain care over the self: a certain form of genetic prudence and genetic responsibility in relation to his or her own life, lifestyle, and marital and reproductive decisions. And of course the norms of prudence and responsibility generate their reverse: That is to say, they enable the identification of those who do not act prudently and responsibly, those who are biologically irresponsible and who may, therefore, be exposed to certain sanctions ranging from disapproval to disentitlement to health services as a result.

BIOMEDICINE: BEYOND TREATMENT AND CURE

In this essay, I have explored the hypothesis that we are inhabiting an "emergent form of life." I have pointed to changing biomedical genomic understandings of our nature as living creatures, in particular ideas of susceptibility and presymptomatic illness, and suggested that human beings themselves are coming to understand their own life form, and with it their rights and responsibilities, their demands, and their obligations, in terms of a new language. Further, I have suggested that the remit of biomedicine now extends beyond the boundaries set by diseases and their treatments, to the management of living in relation to our susceptibilities and the ills that we are at risk of suffering in the future.

Of course, on both these dimensions we are not witnessing something fundamentally new. Individuals have long understood themselves in terms of the language of medicine and have calibrated their lives, made their demands, and felt their responsibilities in terms of the management of a body understood in medical terms. And as we know from innumerable medical histories and critical sociologies, doctors have long exercised power over persons and powers well beyond those concerning frank pathology. We can think of everything from medical concerns with conditions that do not look much like diseases, such as back pain; through medical engagement with women's bodies and reproduction; to the involvement of medicine in such contemporary issues as obesity and baldness; through to the engagement of medical authority since at least the nineteenth century in issues such as town planning and insurance repayments; and, of course, to the whole field of preventive medicine, movements for social and individual hygiene, domestic education, and health promotion. So, what is happening is no epochal shift. But nonetheless I think something new is emerging. The distinction between the treatment of an illness and the management of a condition and the transformation of a form of life is becoming ever more blurred and problematic. This is not limited to ideas of susceptibility and presymptomatic illness. We can see it also where medicine engages with a multitude of intermediate conditions, such as infertility, short stature, and baldness. We can also observe it in relation to variations of mood or conduct occupying a kind of gray area—for example, the expansion of the category of depression, the rise of the anxiety disorders, the spreading diagnosis of attention deficit hyperactivity disorder for troubles of childhood, and the expansion of the use of the diagnosis of "personality disorder" to designate a treatable condition (Rose, 2006). In these diagnoses "on the borderline," the act of diagnosis is closely bound up with the availability of a therapy. That is to say, the expansion of a diagnostic category of depression or personality disorder goes hand in hand with the claims that a particular treatment, in each of these cases a drug treatment, is available to engage with those conditions. Here, to return to a point that I made earlier in this essay, the pathway of medical truth seems to be shaped by the possibilities of generating products that can sell in the market, made possible by these new diagnostic categories.

This link between the act of diagnosis and the availability of therapeutic intervention is not so evident in predictive testing for genomic susceptibilities, where the capacity to gain knowledge of the possible future is, in many cases, in advance of any reliable mode of prophylactic intervention. It is, however, already active in the case of other risk-based medical strategies, such as the use of statins for those with raised blood lipid levels, and it is the dream that inspires many researchers and companies seeking to develop predictive genomic tests. And, from my point of view, what is significant is the emergence of the very idea that the diagnosis of a condition—by means of genomic screening or other tests—that has not yet revealed itself in the actual life of the patient leads to a demand, perhaps even an obligation, for some kind of preventive intervention in relation to it. And this style of thought and action is expanding not just for organic conditions but also for behavioral conditions, especially those of children. It is, perhaps, in this combination of screening, preventive intervention, and in particular the use of pharmaceuticals that one is seeing the most dramatic example of the extension of the powers of biomedicine to the management of life itself (cf. Rose 2001, 2006).

REFERENCES

Fox Keller, Evelyn. 2000. *The century of the gene*. Cambridge, MA: Harvard University Press.
Lock, Margaret. 2005. The eclipse of the gene and the return of divination. *Current Anthropology* 46:S47–S70.
Rabinow, Paul. 1992. Artificiality and enlightenment: From sociobiology to biosociality. In *Incorporations*, edited by J. Crary and S. Kwinter, 234–52. New York: Zone Books.

———. 1996. *Essays on the anthropology of reason.* Princeton, NJ: Princeton University Press.

Rose, Nikolas. 2001. The politics of life itself. *Theory, Culture & Society* 18, no. 6: 1–30.

———. 2006. *The politics of life itself: Biomedicine, power and subjectivity in the twenty-first century.* Princeton, NJ: Princeton University Press.

Rose, Nikolas, and Carlos Novas. 2000. Genetic risk and the birth of the somatic individual. *Economy and Society* 29, no. 4: 485–513.

———. 2004. Biological citizenship. In *Global assemblages: Technology, politics, and ethics as anthropological problems,* edited by Aihwa Ong and Stephen Collier, 439–63. Oxford: Blackwell.

Waldby, Catherine. 2000. *The visible human project: Informatic bodies and post-human medicine.* New York: Routledge.

Susceptible individuals
and risky rights
Dimensions of genetic responsibility

Thomas Lemke

Repeatedly it has been remarked that the results of genomic research are threatening traditional concepts of personal responsibility and individual autonomy. Contemporary biology with its search for genetic (and neurobiological) determinants for a multitude of traits and modes of behavior seems to subvert the substantial basis for responsible action: the possibility of individual decision making and choice.[1] I do not think that this fear of genetic determinism is justified. What we observe today is not the reduction of individual responsibility by reference to genetic dispositions and inborn traits. The discovery of genetic factors that influence and regulate the expression of diseases and personal traits does not result in a position that negates or forecloses the responsibility of the subject; quite the contrary, the increasing genetic knowledge is the central point of reference to expand moral duties. It engenders new modes and fields for responsible action.

In fact, a discourse of genetic responsibility has emerged since the mid-1970s. While genetic responsibility in the 1970s was articulated exclusively in the context of reproductive behavior and referred to the care for "healthy" children and the desire not to transmit "disease genes,"[2] today two other dimensions of responsibility are added. The moral duty for prevention of risk is complemented by obligations to communicate and control genetic risks. First of all, we find an anxiety over possible effects of genetic risks for already living persons: Shouldn't relatives be warned about genetic risks in order to realize options for prevention or therapy? If there are no such options available, shouldn't they know about genetic risks, in order to seek genetic counseling or testing options to make "responsible" decisions concerning their future? There is a second direction in which the discourse of genetic risk has expanded since the 1970s. This new field of application does not concern the relation to others but the health behavior of the person himself or herself. Responsible behavior is expected not only in relation to others, to possible children or existing family members, but also toward one's self in regard to genetic risks. Genetic responsibility in this case is expressed as demand for genetic diagnostics and prevention procedures. As a consequence, only knowledge about individual genetic risks allows for a responsible life.[3] By presenting many diseases as genetic in origin, a "risk-competent" or "rational" health behavior not only demands the acknowledgment of general risk factors like alcohol, smoking, or lack of exercise, but also necessitates a specialized knowledge based on the individual genetic risk profile.[4]

In this essay, I would like to highlight a few dilemmas and problems presented by the discourse of genetic responsibility. Since the focus in the research literature as well as the coverage in the media has been on "responsible parenthood," I will concentrate in this contribution on the two other dimensions of genetic responsibility. My thesis is that the discourse of genetic responsibility tends to undermine guaranteed rights and the freedom of choice concerning genetic tests by establishing imperatives of duty toward oneself and others. First, the duty to inform relatives about their genetic risks may contrast with the protection of privacy and the confidentiality of the doctor–patient relationship. Moreover, the imperative to warn others could erode their right not to know about genetic risks. Second, new forms of discrimination, exclusion, and paternalism might arise in a social and political conjuncture in which genetic information is becoming more and more irresistible. In this social climate it will probably be judged responsible to exclude workers who have been diagnosed as genetically susceptible from health-threatening job positions.

In the following sections, I will concentrate on how the responsibility to communicate and control genetic risks already shapes juridical decisions and how it takes hold in institutional settings such as the patient–physician relationship and in the workplace. I will present several legal cases that were recently decided in the United States, which serve to illustrate that the duty to inform relatives as well as the imperative to control one's own genetic risks are becoming institutionalized.

RIGHT TO NONKNOWLEDGE, OR DUTY TO WARN?

Genetic risks are characterized by a central ambiguity. Genetic information not only concerns the individual but also may indicate health risks for relatives and family. This particular quality of genetic information produces a certain problem: Under what conditions are physicians legally obliged to disclose genetic information that is medically relevant to potentially affected relatives? When do they have to respect the "genetic privacy" of their patients?[5] There are different regulatory frameworks to deal with the problem of confidentiality in the context of genetic information. In France, any direct transmission of genetic information to other persons or institutions is forbidden, while in the United Kingdom and in the United States, as in many other countries, the right of confidentiality is principally guaranteed, but it may be restricted under certain conditions.[6] While all regulations protect the privacy of genetic information, there remains a considerable legal uncertainty when stipulating situations in which such information may be disclosed without liability (Henn 2002; Parker & Lucassen 2002). Two cases in the United States, where high courts ruled that doctors are obliged to warn children of a patient that may be at risk genetically for acquiring the disease of their parent, illustrate a creeping tendency to establish a duty to warn family members about genetic risks. The first case was decided in 1995 by the Florida Supreme Court (*Pate v. Threlkel*, 661 So. 2d 278 [1995]).[7]

The case was brought by Heidi Pate, whose mother was diagnosed with medullary thyroid carcinoma (a presumably inherited tumor) in 1987. After Ms. Pate learned that she had the same disease in 1990, she and her husband sued her mother's physician. The lawsuit alleged that the physician was under a duty to warn the mother of the importance of testing her children for medullary thyroid carcinoma because of its genetic transferability. The plaintiff claimed that had the physician warned her, she would have been tested three years earlier and taken preventive action. The trial court dismissed the plaintiff's claim. It ruled that since Heidi Pate was the patient's daughter, there was no professional relationship with the physician. As a consequence, no substantial ground for bringing a malpractice suit existed. However, since this was the first time such an issue had arisen in Florida, the case was transferred to the Florida Supreme Court.

The Florida Supreme Court in its analysis ruled against the physician. It concluded that the physician's alleged duty to warn extended to the children of the patient even though the children were not his patients:

We conclude that when the prevailing standard of care creates a new duty that is obviously for the benefit of certain identified third parties and the physician knows of the existence of those third parties, then the physician's duty runs to those third parties. (*Pate v. Threlkel* 1995: 282)

The Supreme Court then discussed how the duty could be discharged. For practical reasons and in continuity with professional principles, it ruled that the duty does not require the physician to warn the patient's children of the disease but would be satisfied by warning the patient of the possible health risks for his or her relatives (Petrila 2001: 407–8; Deftos 1998: 964; American Society of Human Genetics [ASHG] 1998: 480).[8]

One year later, a similar case was decided by an appellate court in New Jersey that further extended the professional duties of the physician (*Safer v. Pack*, 677 A.2d 188 [App. Div. NJ, 1996]). In this case the father of the plaintiff, Donna Safer, was treated for cancer in the 1950s and 1960s. He was hospitalized in the beginning of the 1960s for colon cancer and died in 1964 when she was ten years old. In 1990, Donna Safer was diagnosed with colon cancer herself. After obtaining her father's medical records, she filed suit in 1992 against the estate of her father's doctor (who had died in 1969). She alleged that her father's physician knew or should have known of the hereditary nature of the disease, and she saw a violation of a duty to warn her of the risk to her health while her father was treated. According to Safer, a timely warning would have enabled her to take preventive measures to reduce her risk (Petrila 2001: 408–10; Clayton 2003: 566–67).

While the trial court denied the plaintiff's motion of judgment, the appellate court came to another conclusion. Like the Florida Supreme Court before, the New Jersey court concluded that the physician's duty went well beyond the patient to the children themselves. The court held that there is a legal duty to warn those at risk of avoidable harm from genetically transmissible conditions. A very important reason for this judgment was the fact that the court treated genetic risks just like any other type of medical risks, thereby assimilating genetic risks to infection risks. According to the court, there was "no essential difference" between

> the type of genetic threat at issue here and the menace of infection, contagion or threat of physical harm.... The individual at risk is easily identified, and substantial future harm may be averted or minimized by a timely and effective warning. (*Safer v. Pack* 1996: 1192, cited by Petrila 2001: 409)

In this perspective, the transmission of genetic risks by parents appears to be quite similar to the problem of a possible infection, and as there is a duty to warn relatives in the case of contagious diseases, the same must be true for genetic risks. It is the epistemic rapprochement of genetic risk to other forms of medical risk that allows for a normative extension of genetic responsibility.[9]

But, as the ASHG correctly remarked, the contagious-disease model "is not an ideal paradigm for the disclosure of genetic information" (ASHG 1998: 477).[10] There are several substantial differences between genetic risks and infection risks: The first concerns the etiology of the disease. While genetic conditions are transmitted "vertically through succeeding generations...contagious disease is generally transmitted horizontally...and its impact on others occurs through some form of contact." In contrast to infection risks, genetic risks cannot be separated from the person herself or himself; they are not temporary and accidental, but an integral part of the physical constitution. The second difference concerns the type of intervention. Contagious disease is "controlled by isolation of infected people, by avoidance of whatever contact causes infection, or by cure. Genetic conditions, on the other hand, are controlled not only through prevention or palliative treatment but also through reproductive decisions and choices" (ASHG 1998: 477). There is a third difference that points to the consequences of the analogy between infection risks and genetic risks: Warning relatives about genetic risks will not prevent them from having the gene (Andrews 1997: 268–69).

The two court decisions institutionalize a legal duty of the physician to warn if he or she knows or should have known that the patient's children are exposed to a genetic risk that is related to the disease diagnosed in the patient. In both cases, it was held that there are legal obligations that go beyond the concrete relationship between the physician and his or her patients toward the patient's children. This tendency to establish a duty to warn in the context of genetically transmissible diseases results in some serious problems.[11] First, it might be asked if the establishment of such a duty of disclosure does not undermine the right not to know about genetic risks. Probably, there are family members who do not want to be warned of their increased genetic risks. How is it possible to exercise a right not to know if the doctor is legally obliged to inform the relatives? As a consequence, the often cited right not to know about genetic information might lack any substance in a society that gives priority to unconditioned information and that assumes that responsible persons are only those who actively seek genetic information. This reasoning is stated quite clearly in a report on genetic screening that was published by the Nuffield Council on Bioethics:

> As a starting point, we adopt the view that a person acting responsibly would normally wish to communicate important genetic information to other family members who may have an interest in that information, and that a responsible person would normally wish to receive that information, particularly where it may have a bearing on decisions which he or she may be called upon to take in the future. (Nuffield Council on Bioethics 1993: 49)[12]

Let me just mention some more problems that will arise in the context of a medical duty to warn relatives of genetic risks. The disclosure of this kind of information may have negative effects on family relations and lead to severe tensions between family members (D'Agincourt-Canning 2001; Finkler et al. 2003). Also, the genetic information might be used by third parties. Employers and insurance companies are certainly interested in this kind of information, and there is a danger that it will be used for discriminative purposes (Billings et al. 1992; Lemke 2006b).

A DIRECT THREAT: SUSCEPTIBILITY, PATERNALISM, AND DISCRIMINATION

This brings me to the third court decision that I would like to present: the *Chevron v. Echazabal* case that was decided by the U.S. Supreme Court in 2002. The plaintiff, Mario Echazabal, had worked at a Chevron oil refinery in El Segundo, California since 1972, as a laborer, helper, and pipe fitter for various contractors, mainly in the coker unit. In 1992, he applied to work directly for Chevron at the refinery's coker unit. Chevron determined that Echazabal was qualified for the job and offered to hire him contingent on the results of a physical exam. The company doctor, however, declared

Echazabal unfit for the job because blood tests showed liver abnormality. During the examination, a liver function assay was used that resulted in the identification of a biological marker that, according to the employer, disposed Echazabal for liver impairment. As a consequence, he would face further damage if he experienced chemical exposures characteristic of refinery work. Nonetheless, Echazabal was permitted to continue working at the company as an employee of Chevron's contractor. He sought treatment and was ultimately diagnosed with hepatitis C that has remained asymptomatic since then. In 1995, he again applied for a job at Chevron, and again his demand was turned down after a medical exam. This time, the company directed the contractor who employed Echazabal to take him out of that position, which it did in 1996. This action was taken even though Echazabal's liver condition never caused injury or accident to himself or anyone else at the refinery. In 1997, he filed suit, charging that Chevron's decision violated the Americans with Disabilities Act (ADA). He also presented testimony by two medical experts in liver disease that working in that factory would not put him at any greater risk than any other employee. Chevron defended itself under a regulation of the Equal Employment Opportunity Commission permitting the defense that a worker's disability on the job would pose a "direct threat" (*Chevron v. Echazabal* 2002: 1–3; National Council on Disability [NCD] 2003: 5–6).

After a district court granted summary judgment for Chevron and a circuit court reversed this decision, the case was presented to the U.S. Supreme Court. The Supreme Court addressed in its decision issues central to the ADA. At the heart of the ruling is the court's interpretation of the "direct threat" provision of the ADA since an individual may be refused employment if a direct threat can be established. The previous ruling in this case by a circuit court held that the direct threat defense was not available to Chevron because Echazabal only presented a risk to himself. According to the court, a "direct threat" only applies when the individual's condition poses a direct threat to others. In this perspective, health is conceived as a "discretionary right in which the individual may choose to assume certain risks so long as they do not have the potential to harm others" (Lomax 2002: A505). This reasoning was rejected and reversed by the Supreme Court. The court held that individuals who pose a risk exclusively to themselves may be excluded from a job as long as the employer relies on "reasonable medical judgment" (*Chevron v. Echazabal* 2002: 12). The company thereby sought to "protect" an individual such as Echazabal from himself.

By presenting evidence from a biological marker, Chevron relied on a medical opinion that is based on future possibilities. The same is true for genetic susceptibility testing. Since the ADA is often cited as offering individuals protection from genetic discrimination, one might ask the (speculative) question if the decision would have been different in this case. According to the Supreme Court, it is acceptable to exclude individuals from a job who pose a risk exclusively to themselves as long as the employer relies "on the most current medical knowledge and/or the best available objective evidence" (*Chevron v. Echazabal* 2002: 12). This condition might be fulfilled by genetic susceptibility testing that increasingly acquires medical and scientific credibility. As a consequence, it is conceivable that future workplace exclusion might be based on the diagnosis of genetic susceptibilities. The Supreme Court decision might be important for the "asymptomatic ill" (Billings et al. 1992), as the National Council on Disability (NCD), an independent federal agency that was instrumental in creating the legislative record that Congress considered in enacting the ADA, predicts: "With advances in medical technology, including genetic screening, there also is the potential for excluding large numbers of pre-symptomatic individuals (i.e. 'the healthy ill') on the basis of potential health or safety risks to themselves in the future" (NCD 2003: 11; see also Lomax 2002).

The court decision denies employees the right to decide whether or not to accept the risks posed by a particular job and reinstates a paternalistic logic that says that the company knows what's best for the employee or potential employee. Ironically, it was exactly this paternalistic logic that should have been abandoned by the ADA regulation. Therefore, the NCD sees in the court decision a reversal of the original intentions of the law:

> Congress acknowledged in the ADA that discrimination takes many forms, including paternalism and stereotyping. Perhaps the most long-standing and insidious aspect of this type of discrimination is the assumption that people with disabilities are not competent to make informed, wise, or safe life choices. (NCD 2003: 9)

The NCD argues that the decision will make it much easier for employers in the United States to exclude workers by referring to the possibility of a direct threat that originates in a higher genetic susceptibility—a trend already visible in recent court decisions (see NCD 2003: 15–16).

Apart from its effect on disability rights, the *Chevron v. Echazabal* decision may have important implications for environmental health research (Lomax 2002: A504). While research in this field traditionally concentrated on identifying external risk factors that pose health problems to employees, more and more scientific emphasis is put on recognizing internal risks or personal susceptibilities that are based on the genetic makeup of individuals. As a consequence the "old" risk logic is completely reversed. The scientific interest no longer focuses on bad working conditions or toxic substances that are used in the labor process but on "supersensitive workers" (Daniels 2003: 548) or susceptible employees who are less resistant than others to environmental risk factors and health-threatening conditions of work.

This tendency is illustrated by a case that involved a railway company in the United States. In 2001, it came to light that Burlington Northern Santa Fe Railway (BNSF) began obtaining blood for DNA testing from employees who were seeking disability compensation as a result of carpal tunnel syndrome that occurred at the job. The employees were not told the purpose of the tests, which was to detect a mutation that is associated with the disease. Though the motive remained unclear, "it seems reasonable to suspect that BNSF would have tried to deny disability benefits to any employee who had such a mutation, arguing that the mutation, and not the job, caused carpal tunnel syndrome" (Clayton 2003: 563; Lehming 2001).[13]

Since there are more and more genetic tests for different conditions available, there is a real danger that employers might use genetic information to determine how "genetically fit" someone is for a job. Already in 1997, a survey by the American Management Association showed that 6 to 10 percent of employers were conducting genetic testing (Dearing 2002: 8). But the problem is not limited to the United States. In the United Kingdom, current laws allow employers to refuse someone a job on the basis of their genetic testing results (GeneWatch UK 2003). In Germany, the federal government is discussing a law that would permit genetic testing for employees in jobs like public transportation or construction for symptoms of color-blindness, among other things—even if it remains unclear what the use of genetic testing for something symptomatic would be (Tzorzis 2004; Nationaler Ethikrat 2005).[14]

CONCLUSION: THE EMERGENCE OF A GENETIC ENLIGHTENMENT

This brief discussion illustrates some problems and dilemmas that are brought about by the new genetics and the increasing possibilities of genetic testing. I argued that we observe a discourse of genetic responsibility that goes beyond bioethical considerations and is already shaping legal decisions. Furthermore, I distinguished three dimensions of genetic responsibility. First, genetic responsibility concerns reproductive decisions to prevent disease and disability in the next generation. Genetic responsibility in this context means to act in such a way as to guarantee the birth of healthy children and to prevent the transmission of "faulty" genes. Since the 1970s, genetics was increasingly introduced into medical practice, especially in the field of diagnosis. In the United States and other industrialized states, genetic knowledge was used in screening programs for certain diseases, new reproductive technologies were developed, and prenatal diagnosis became part of medical care for pregnant women (Duster 1990; Rapp 2000). As an increasing number of women are now offered prenatal testing and tests for more and more conditions, giving birth to a disabled child seems to be a matter of choice rather than fate. It appears to be more a blameworthy failure of surveillance and control than an unfortunate piece of bad luck. As Professor Robert Edwards, the pioneer of in vitro fertilization (IVF), has put it, "In the future, it will be a sin to have a disabled child" (cited by Shakespeare 2003: 205).

Second, genetic responsibility means the obligation to warn family members of genetic risks. This new dimension of responsibility refers to the communication of genetic risks. To transmit genetic information to relatives is seen as an important indicator for a well-ordered and functioning family life, as a test for responsible thinking and care for each other, and as a symbol of superior moral quality. As a genetic counselor wrote,

> Each of us has the ethical responsibility to communicate vital information to our relatives…. Hiding the truth behind a cover of concern for the feelings of individual family members is unacceptable when the wellness and the very life of another [are] at stake. We have a moral imperative to tell. (Milunsky 2001: 7)[15]

Third, genetic responsibility is increasingly addressed to the individual, as responsibility toward the self. It means control of diseases by the prudent management of genetic risks through informed choices of lifestyle options that are based on genetic information. Genetic responsibility here means the active demand for genetic information and the interest in genetic testing opportunities. This scenario is well described by a hypothetical case that is presented by Francis Collins, director of the National Human Genome Research Institute of the United States:

> John, a 23-year-old college graduate, is referred to his physician because a serum cholesterol level of 255 mg per deciliter was detected in the course of a medical examination required for employment…. To obtain more precise information about his risks of contracting coronary artery disease and other illnesses in the future, John agrees to consider a battery of genetic tests that are available in 2010. After working through an interactive computer program that explains the benefits and risks of such tests, John agrees…to undergo 15 genetic tests that provide risk information for illnesses for which preventive strategies are available…. A cheek-swab DNA specimen is sent off for testing, and the results are returned in one week. John's subsequent counselling session with the physician and a genetic nurse specialist focuses on the conditions for which his risk differs substantially (by a factor of more than two) from that of the general population…. John is pleased to learn that genetic testing does not always give bad news—his risks of contracting prostate cancer and Alzheimer's disease are reduced, because he carries low-risk variants of the several genes known in 2010 to contribute to these illnesses. But John is sobered by the evidence of his increased risks of contracting coronary artery disease, colon cancer, and lung cancer. Confronted with the reality of his own genetic data, he arrives at that crucial "teachable moment" when a lifelong change in health-related

behavior...is possible.... His risk of colon cancer can be addressed by
beginning a program of annual colonoscopy at the age of 45, which
in his situation is a very cost-effective way to avoid colon cancer. His
substantial risk of contracting lung cancer provides the key motivation
for him to join a support group of persons at genetically high risk for
serious complications of smoking, and he successfully kicks the habit.
(Collins 1999: 34–35)[16]

The fictive example clearly demonstrates that the proliferation of genetic
knowledge and testing devices does not abolish individual responsibility and
choice; it rather produces, if seemingly paradoxically, a new form of autonomous subjectivity. The individual is conceived not as a passive recipient
of medical advice, but as an active seeker of information and consumer of
genetic testing devices and health care services (Petersen & Bunton 2002).
The social significance of genome analysis and genetic diagnostics lies less
in the factual deterministic relationship that they seem to offer, and more
in the "reflexive" relationship that they generate between an individual risk
profile and social requirements.[17] Bioethicist Hans-Martin Sass therefore
calls for an "ethos of duty" in handling genetic information:

Leisure time behavior, place of work, or genetic predisposition, or a
mixture of all three factors determine[s] the respective individual risks
to my health.... Some can be eliminated, others reduced, or the stage at
which they become acute delayed. The patient becomes the partner in
preventing or delaying major health risks. The doctor's ethics under the
Hippocratic oath, that is characterized by care and outer-determined
support, will in future be complemented by a self-determined and self-
responsible ethics of the patient and citizen in healthcare. (Sass 1994:
343; transl. TL)

Nevertheless, the autonomy in question relies on a rather specific and
liberal conception of morality. It is limited insofar as the individual is considered an abstract subject free from material restrictions, cultural values,
and social bonds. He or she is forced to choose between an array of pre-
established options and to take responsibility for the consequences of his
or her choices. Only those actors who accept health as a superior social
and moral value and who regard biomedical and scientific expertise as
essential for everyday life and personal decision making qualify as rational
or responsible subjects (Callon & Rabeharisoa 2004; Beeson & Doksum
2001). This genetic enlightenment (or "literacy") entails a precise notion
of *Mündigkeit* (maturity), which is linked to possessing adequate medical
information and to the knowledge of one's genetic risks (Sass 2003). It contributes to constituting a "homo geneticus" (Gaudillière 1995: 35; Novas &
Rose 2000) who submits to practices of self-control and personal manage-

ment of the body—which comprises an embodiment of risk technologies and genetic knowledge.

The reference to personal responsibility and self-determination only makes sense if the individual is more than a victim or prisoner of her or his genetic material. If there is indeed a direct relationship between genotype and phenotype in the sense of genetic determinism, then it would be far harder to uphold the appeal to individual autonomy. By contrast, the construction of "at-risk" individuals, families, and pregnancies makes it easier to moralize on deviant behavior and to assign guilt and responsibility (Douglas 1990). Paradoxically, it is exactly the invitation to engage in self-determination and the imperative of a "genetic responsibility" that render individuals more and more dependent on medico-scientific authorities and their information. The right to health is realized in the form of duty to procure information, and only those who act responsibly draw the correct, that is, risk-minimizing and forward-oriented, conclusions from this range of information.

NOTES

Acknowledgment. A previous version of this chapter was presented at the Vital Politics Conference, London School of Economics and Political Science, September 5–7, 2003.

1. See for example Dan W. Brock's observation that the Human Genome Project is likely to affect deeply...our conception of ourselves as responsible agents and, more specifically, as morally and legally responsible for our actions, for the lives we live, and for the kinds of people that we become. (1999: 23)
2. For example, Hardin (1974: 88):
   We must admit that if there is one thing a person is not responsible for, it is the genes that were passed on him.... We are not responsible as the recipients of errors. But should we not be responsible as the transmitters of errors? If there are some people in society who refuse to take such responsibility, who say *No* for whatever reason, refusing to inhibit their own breeding in spite of the fact they are passing on genes known to be undesirable genes, does not then the issue of responsibility arise in a very acute form?... Should individual freedom include the freedom to impose upon society costs that society does not want?... We must recognize that this is a finite world. The money we spend for one purpose, we cannot spend on another.
   See also Twiss (1974) and Lebel (1977).
3. For a conceptual exploration of "genetic irresponsibility," see Andre et al. (2000).
4. Anne Kerr and Tom Shakespeare (2002: 153–54) likewise distinguish two sorts of responsibility that individuals bear who are found to be at risk for a genetic disease: "The first is to avoid behaviours likely to exacerbate that risk. This starts with consulting and following the advice of medical experts.... Second, individuals bear responsibility for informing their genetic kin about their risk." The extension of the discourse of genetic responsibility from the

focus on reproduction to the interest in communication and control of genetic risks can be empirically demonstrated by an analysis of medical advice books and self-help manuals from the 1970s onwards (Lemke 2006a, 2006b).

5. On the question of "genetic privacy," see the contributions in Rothstein (1997). For the German discussion, see Meyer (2001: 102–42) and Damm (2003).

6. See for example the statement of the American Society of Human Genetics:
    Disclosure should be permissible where attempts to encourage disclosure on the part of the patient have failed; where the harm is highly likely to occur and is serious and foreseeable; where the at-risk relative(s) is identifiable; and where either the disease is preventable/treatable or medically accepted standards indicate that early monitoring will reduce the genetic risk. (ASHG 1998: 474)

7. The professional obligation that physicians could be liable to persons with whom they have never established a patient–physician relationship was stated in a prior lawsuit (*Tarasoff et al. v. The Regents of the University of California et al.* 1976 [17 Cal.3d 425]). On prior lawsuits in which the issue of information on genetic risks was raised, see Andrews (1997: 266–73). For an overview on the duty of physicians to warn the relatives of their patients of the presence of genetic disease in the family as an evolving area of the law of medicine in the United States, see Deftos (1998).

8. From *Pate v. Threlkel* (1995: 282):
    The patient ordinarily can be expected to pass on the warning. To require the physician to seek out and warn various members of the patient's family would often be difficult or impractical and would place too heavy a burden upon the physician. Thus, we emphasize that in any circumstances in which the physician has a duty to warn of a genetically transferable disease, that duty will be satisfied by warning the patient.

9. According to Peter Conrad, the paradigm of molecular medicine does not replace but actually relies on bacteriological conceptions of disease:
    In my view, the close fit between germ theory and gene theory is one of the chief reasons that genetic explanations have been so readily accepted in medicine and the popular discourse. At least on the level of assumptions and structure, gene theory does not challenge common conceptions of aetiology but rather shifts its focus. In this sense at least, genetics is a complementary rather than a challenging paradigm in medicine. (Conrad 1999: 232; see also Steinberg 1996)

10. The following distinction draws on the argument in the ASHG statement (1998).

11. For a more comprehensive elaboration, see Petrila (2001: 415–18).

12. Jorgen Husted has convincingly demonstrated that a legal duty to warn not only effectively eliminates the right of nonknowledge but also breaks with the professional principle of nondirectiveness in counseling on medical options and renews medical paternalism:
    Thus the unsolicited disclosure, whether by the relative following the doctor's strong suggestion or by the doctor acting independently, seems to be a clear cut case of strong medical paternalism—acting solely from the medical point of view the decision "To know or not to know?" is taken out of the hands of the unsuspecting individual, for her or his own good of course. (Husted 1997: 57)

13. For more case material on genetic discrimination in the workplace, see Martindale (2001), Miller (1998), and Marshall (1999).

14. An early discussion of this problem in Germany is presented in Klees (1990, 1992); for a more recent analysis, see Zinke (2003). For a critique of current developments in France, see Thébaud Mondy (1999).

15. For an empirical illustration of this dimension of responsibility in the context of predictive testing for "breast cancer genes," see Hallowell (1999).
16. For a similar scenario, see the Internet publication "Your Genes, Your Choices," by the American Association for the Advancement of Science (2003) that emphasizes the importance of "genetic literacy." Actually, the future seems to be pretty close, since it is already possible to get individual genome scans; see Kristof (2003) for a description of that experience.
17. For an elaboration of this argument, see Lemke (2004).

REFERENCES

American Association for the Advancement of Science. 2003. Your genes, your choices. http://www.ornl.gov/TechResources/Human_Genome/publicat/genechoice/contents.html (accessed November 9, 2006).

American Society of Human Genetics Social Issues Subcommittee on Familial Disclosure. 1998. ASHG statement: Professional disclosure of familial genetic information. *American Journal of Human Genetics* 62:474–83.

Andre, Judith, Leonhard M. Fleck, and Tom Tomlinson. 2000. On being genetically "irresponsible." *Kennedy Institute of Ethics Journal* 10, no. 2: 129–46.

Andrews, Lori B. 1997. Gen-etiquette: Genetic information, family relationships, and adoption. In *Genetic secrets: Protecting privacy and confidentiality in the genetic era*, edited by M. A. Rothstein, 255–80. New Haven, CT: Yale University Press.

Beeson, Diane, and Teresa Doksum. 2001. Family values and resistance to genetic testing. In *Bioethics in social context*, edited by B. Hoffmaster, 153–78. Philadelphia: Temple University Press.

Billings, Paul, et al. 1992. Discrimination as a consequence of genetic testing. *American Journal of Human Genetics* 50:476–82.

Brock, Dan W. 1999. The Human Genome Project and human identity. In *Genes and human self-knowledge: Historical and philosophical reflections on modern genetics*, edited by Robert F. Weir, Susan C. Lawrence, and Evan Fales, 18–33. Iowa City: University of Iowa Press.

Callon, Michel, and Vololona Rabeharisoa. 2004. Gino's lesson on humanity: Genetics, mutual entanglements and the sociologist's rule. *Economy and Society* 33:1–27.

Chevron USA, Inc. v. Echazabel, 122 S. Ct. 2045 (2002).

Clayton, Ellen Wright. 2003. Ethical, legal, and social implications of genomic medicine. *New England Journal of Medicine* 349:562–69.

Collins, Francis S. 1999. Shattuck lecture: Medical and societal consequences of the Human Genome Project. *New England Journal of Medicine* 341:28–37.

Conrad, Peter. 1999. A mirage of genes. *Sociology of Health & Illness* 21: 228–41.

D'Agincourt-Canning, Lori. 2001. Experiences of genetic risk: Disclosure and the gendering of responsibility. *Bioethics* 15, no. 3: 231–47.

Damm, Reinhard. 2003. Prädiktive genetische Tests: Gesellschaftliche Folgen und rechtlicher Schutz der Persönlichkeit. In *Das genetische Wissen und die Zukunft des Menschen*, edited by L. Honnefelder et al., 203–28. Berlin: Walter de Gruyter.

Daniels, Norman. 2003. *Chevron v Echazabal*: Protection, opportunity, and paternalism. *American Journal of Public Health* 93:545–48.

Dearing, Ann. 2002. Genetic discrimination. *Risk Management* (July): 8–9.

Deftos, Leonard J. 1998. The evolving duty to disclose the presence of genetic disease to relatives. *Academic Medicine* 73:962–68.

Douglas, Mary. 1990. Risk as a forensic resource. *Daedalus* 119:1–16.

Duster, Troy. 1990. *Backdoor to eugenics*. New York: Routledge.

Finkler, Kaja, Cécile Skrzynia, and James P. Evans. 2003. The new genetics and its consequences for family, kinship, medicine and medical genetics. *Social Science and Medicine* 57:403–12.

Gaudillière, Jean-Paul. 1995. Sequenzieren, Zählen und Vorhersehen. Praktiken einer Genverwaltung. *Tüte* (special issue, "Wissen und Macht—Die Krise des Regierens, Tübingen"): 34–39.

GeneWatch UK. 2003. *Genetic testing in the workplace: Creating a genetic underclass?* Report Briefing no. 24. London: GeneWatch UK.

Hallowell, Nina. 1999. Doing the right thing: Genetic risk and responsibility. In *Sociological Perspectives on the New Genetics*, edited by P. Conrad and J. Gabe, 97–120. Oxford: Blackwell.

Hardin, Garrett. 1974. The moral threat of personal medicine. In *Genetic responsibility: On choosing our children's genes*, edited by Mack Lipkin Jr. and Peter T. Rowley, 85–91. New York: Plenum Press.

Henn, Wolfram. 2002. Probleme der ärztlichen Schweigepflicht in Familien mit Erbkrankheiten. *Zeitschrift für Medizinische Ethik* 48:343–54.

Husted, Jorgen. 1997. Autonomy and a right not to know. In *The right to know and the right not to know*, edited by Ruth Chadwick, Mairi Levitt, and Darren Shickle, 55–68. Aldershot, UK: Avebury.

Kerr, Anne, and Tom Shakespeare. 2002. *Genetic politics: From eugenics to genome*. Oxford: New Clarion Press.

Klees, Bernd. 1990. *Der Griff in die Erbanlagen. Verdrängte Probleme der Genomanalyse*. Braunschweig: Steinweg Verlag.

———. 1992. Schöne neue Welt—oder neuer Sozialdarwinismus? Auswirkungen von Bio- und Gentechnologien auf die Arbeitswelt. In *Lebensqualität statt Qualitätskontrolle menschlichen Lebens*, edited by A-D. Stein, 199–250. Berlin: Marhold.

Kristof, Nicholas D. 2003. Staying alive, staying human. *New York Times*, February 11.

Lebel, Robert R. 1977. Approach to notion of genetic responsibility. *American Journal of Human Genetics* 29, no. 6: A67.

Lehming, Malte. 2001. US-Unternehmen wegen Gentests verklagt. *Der Tagesspiegel*, February 12, 5.

Lemke, Thomas. 2004. Disposition and determinism: Genetic diagnostics in risk society. *The Sociological Review* 52:550–66.

———. 2006a. Genetic responsibility and neo-liberal governmentality: Medical diagnosis as moral terrain. In *Michel Foucault and Power Today. International Multidisciplinary Studies in the History of the Present*, edited by Alain Beaulieu and David Gabbard, 83–91. Lanham, MD: Lexington Books.

———. 2006b. *Die Polizei der Gene. Formen und Felder genetischer Diskriminierung*, Frankfurt am Main: Campus.

Lomax, Geoffrey. 2002. *Chevron v. Echazabal*: A sobering decision for environmental health research. *Environmental Health Perspectives* 110, no. 9: A504–A505.

Marshall, Eliot. 1999. Beryllium screening raises ethical issues. *Science* 285:178–79.

Martindale, Diane. 2001. Pink slip in your genes. *Scientific American*, no. 1: 13–14.

Meyer, Ingo 2001. *"Der Mensch als Datenträger?" Zur verfassungsrechtlichen Bewertung postnataler genetischer Untersuchungen*. Berlin: Berlin Verlag.

Miller, Paul Steven. 1998. Genetic discrimination in the workplace. *Journal of Law, Medicine and Ethics* 26:189–97.

Milunsky, Aubrey. 2001. *Your genetic destiny: Know your genes, secure your health, save your life.* Cambridge, MA: Perseus.

National Council on Disability (NCD). 2003. *Chevron v. Echazabal*: The ADA's "direct threat to self." Policy Brief Series: Righting the ADA, no. 9, February 27. http://www.ncd.gov/newsroom/publications/pdf/directthreat.pdf (accessed November 9, 2006).

Nationaler Ethikrat, ed. 2005. *Prädiktive Gesundheitsinformationen bei Einstellungsuntersuchungen.* Berlin: Nationaler Ethikrat.

Novas, Carlos, and Nikolas Rose. 2000. Genetic risk and the birth of the somatic individual. *Economy and Society* 29, no. 4: 485–513.

Nuffield Council on Bioethics. 1993. *Genetic screening. Ethical issues.* London: Nuffield Council on Bioethics.

Parker, Michael, and Anneke. Lucassen. 2002. Working towards ethical management of genetic testing. *The Lancet* 360:1685–87.

Pate v. Threlkel. 661 So. 2d 278 (1995).

Petersen, Alan, and Robin Bunton. 2002. *The new genetics and the public's health.* London: Routledge.

Petrila, John. 2001. Genetic risk: The new frontier for the duty to warn. *Behavioral Sciences & the Law* 19:405–21.

Rapp, Rayna. 2000. *Testing women, testing the fetus: The social impact of amniocentesis in America.* New York: Routledge.

Rothstein, Mark A. 1997. *Genetic secrets: Protecting privacy and confidentiality in the genetic era.* New Haven, CT: Yale University Press.

Safer v. Pack. 677 A.2d 188 (App. Div. NJ, 1996).

Sass, Hans-Martin. 1994. Der Mensch im Zeitalter von genetischer Diagnostik und Manipulation. Kultur, Wissen und Verantwortung. In *Wieviel Genetik braucht der Mensch? Die alten Träume der Genetiker und ihre heutigen Methoden*, edited by Ernst Peter Fischer and Erhard Geißler, 339–53. Konstanz: Universitätsverlag Konstanz.

———. 2003. Patienten- und Bürgeraufklärung über genetische Risikofaktoren. In *Patientenaufklärung bei genetischem Risiko*, edited by Hans-Martin Sass and Peter Schröder, 41–55. Münster u.a.: Lit-Verlag.

Shakespeare, Tom. 2003. Rights, risks and responsibilities: New genetics and disabled people. In *Debating biology: Sociological reflections on health, medicine and society*, edited by S. J. Williams, L. Birke, and G. A. Bendelow, 198–209. London: Routledge.

Steinberg, Deborah Lynn. 1996. Languages of risk: Genetic encryptions of the female body. *Women: A Cultural Review* 7:259–70.

Tarasoff et al. v. The Regents of the University of California et al. 17 Cal.3d 425 (1976).

Thébaud Mondy, Annie. 1999. Genetische Diskriminierung am Arbeitsplatz. *Le Monde Diplomatique*, May 14, 7.

Twiss, Sumner B. 1974. Ethical issues in genetic screening: Models of genetic responsibility. In *Ethical, social and legal dimensions of screening for human genetic disease*, edited by Daniel Bergsma, 225–61. New York: Stratton Intercontinental Medical.

Tzorzis, Andreas. 2004. Are you (genetically) up to the job? *Deutsche Welle* 25 (October):   http://www.dw-world.de/dw/article/0,1564,1369432,00.html (accessed October 26, 2004).

Zinke, Eva. 2003. Der gläserne Mensch in der Arbeitswelt. *Gen-Ethischer Informationsdienst* 19, no. 158: 23–25.

10 "Pop genes"

An investigation of "the gene" in popular parlance

Barbara Duden and Silja Samerski

"POP GENES" AS AN ANALOGY TO THE FLESH: THE ALCHEMICAL POWER OF "GENES" IN ORDINARY SPEECH

Since the mid-1980s, the word *gene* has migrated from science into ordinary conversations. Gene talk has spread epidemically in political and professional arguments and ethical debates, but references to "genes" have also surreptitiously entered personal deliberations. "Genes" by now reshape not only political, social, or medical concepts, but also the very perception of the self. This intrusion of the term into common parlance, and particularly the drastic encroachment of "genes" into personal deliberation—where "genes" have come to impose themselves as the ultimate answer to such primordial questions as "Where do I come from, who am I, and what will happen to me in the future?"—stimulated our curiosity and led to the research project that we report on here. In this chapter, we will first describe the outlines of our investigation and then attempt to make a hypothesis plausible: In the shadow of human genetics, the first person singular, the "I" of the speaker, is subtly, profoundly, and quite probably irreversibly affected. This transformation is not carried through by a series of findings emanating from human genetic research in biomedical laboratories or clinical practice but through the symbolic fallout of gene talk. At the core of this transformation of the embodied "ego" lies—so we observed—an exceptional transformative power of the term when it migrates into ordinary prose. "Genes" in ordinary speech have all that it takes to perform a blending together or superimposition of incompatible spheres of meaning: the word conflates the concrete and abstract, visible and invisible, tangible and conjectured, individual and statistical, and past, present, and future. This alchemistic potency of the term when it appears in ordinary prose has endowed it with the capacity to exercise a crucial symbolic social function in the epochal transformation since the 1980s: The "gene" in ordinary prose imparts bodily substance to the nature of personhood that corresponds to the risk society, in which actuarial calculations and reasoning about the human have become pervasive. This is why parlance about human genetics offers a privileged instance from which to study the uprooting of commonsense perception in the present moment of history.

THE "POP GENE" PROJECT: IN SEARCH OF THE SEMANTIC CONTOURS OF THE "REFLEXIVE GENE"

For almost three years, we have collaborated on an investigation of the quotidian or "pop" gene, pursuing a precise and specific goal: to analyze the meanings of the terms *gene* and *genetic* when they appear in ordinary German prose. Both of us brought discrete experiences to this investigation: One of us is a historian who has learned to distance herself from contemporary certainties by studying women's complaints made in a physician's practice in the early eighteenth century (Duden 1991).[1] She forged methods to grasp past carnal self-reference and called these "historical somatics." Her earlier historical work demanded a self-critical reflection on stance and distance. Critical distance is required for "historical somatics" no less than for the scrutiny of the late twentieth-century disembodiment of the senses that has deepened under the aegis of genetics. The other author is a geneticist and social scientist who has previously studied the effect of laboratory language in everyday life. Taking the example of genetic counseling, she investigated what is demanded from people when they are asked to make decisions in the shadow of laboratory constructs such as "chromosomes," "genes," and "genetic risk." She argues that genetic counseling is paradigmatic of a new form of professional tutelage, namely, the attempt to transform people into managerial decision makers on their own behalf (Samerski 2002, 2005). Understandings of both bygone apperceptions and contemporary human genetics in the laboratory as well as in educational settings were thus conjoined to focus on one question: What are the semantic and praxeological contours of that which people refer to in ordinary conversations as "genes"?

We soon realized that the word *gene* in colloquial speech acts has two particular characteristics: The term is reflexive, pointing back to the speaker, and it implies a somatic deixis, referring to something carnal, something corporeal, something substantial in the person. Because the word *gene* has this reflexive deictic—appointing—power, the speaker's soma, the stuff she or he is made of, turns into something made of genes. In the course of our research, we became aware that the "gene" in ordinary speech is a term with a transformative power unlike that of any other word: It reinterprets the speaker in his or her very flesh. Each mention of the "gene" for the speaker or the addressed equals an alchemical fusion: The "reflexive gene" performs a synthesis of genotype and phenotype; it merges an underlying instance and the soma. This four-letter word's remarkable characteristics, its capacity to perform a shortcut between genotype and phenotype through conversations about genes, merited an investigation.

The perceptual, reflexive, and somatic consequences of references to genetics have barely provoked comment in the vast literature on the cultural impact of genetics. Researchers quite often take "genes" for granted, and preclude the term from analysis as an unquestionable given.[2] Thus, we decided to follow the road less traveled. Here we do not seek to investigate laypeople's "understanding" or "misunderstanding" of genetics; such a frame always precluded analysis of a "something" that the layperson either understood "correctly" or "incorrectly." Yet it was exactly this "something" that we decided to move to the center of our focus: What is the "referent" of gene talk in popular parlance, given the reflexive deictic characteristic of the term? How can we explore the semantic and praxeological contours of that which is evoked with this term? We have coined a neologism to denote this "something," calling it the "pop gene." Our research thus focused on "something" that is precise yet elusive: the "appointing power," that which is implicit in conversations on "genes." The goal of our research was strictly delimited, yet the object of investigation deliberately undefined: the semantic and praxeological contours of "genes" as these take shape in ordinary speech.

"GENES" VIVA VOCE

Equipped with the insights mentioned above—the reflexive, deictic, and somatic characteristic of the word—we were convinced that the question under investigation could not be explored through discourse analysis, that is, through analysis of references to "genes" in the written form. It became clear that our avenue for tracing the implicit or explicit meanings in gene talk lay in ordinary parlance, everyday speech and conversation. We had to concentrate on particular oral situations in which "genes" are mentioned, spoken, and heard about. Somebody must speak to another person about "genes" and expect that the listener understands what is being said as meaningful.

This focus on an "oral gene" proved to be of critical importance. Why? In addressing another person face to face, the speaker usually tries to give meaning to his or her words, and he or she aims to be understood by the listener. When we speak to another person, we certainly make an effort not to speak indecipherable gibberish: We want to say something meaningful to the listener because we are addressing him or her. Speaking to a concrete person—voiced utterance addressed to listening ears—anchors those utterances to the realm of commonsense perception and understanding.

A second insight strengthened our insistence on studying the reflexive, deictic, and semantic contours of an "oral gene." By talking about "genes," speakers inevitably talk about their corporeal substance; they refer to the body they assume they have. In recent years, people have gotten used to addressing themselves and others as instances of technogene constructs; when one refers to his or her mind as a backup system, one incorporates information processing, and the distality—the chasm between the referent of the predication and the somatic being of the speaker—gets obscured. In oral speech, the abyss between the technogene referent and the concrete living speaker becomes more evident than in written texts, for the heterogeneity of the technical and the personal is more likely to be intuitively recognized in oral intercourse. This is also true when somebody transforms her embodied personal "ego" into a "case" to which statistics, probabilities, and population management adhere: The sensual, perceptual presence that has been elided with mathematical calculations still resonates. In oral, commonsense conversation, "genes" dramatically enact the disturbing fusion of flesh and blood with statistical constructs.

In relying on the heuristic fruitfulness of listening to a speaker rather than "reading" the "body" from textual descriptions, we follow the method of Ruth Padel, a classicist, who insisted in a brilliant analysis of early Greek medical and theatrical texts about the self that these can only be fully grasped by being voiced. "I am not treating their work as theory, as the object of analysis," she writes, referring to the Pre-Socratics' embodied self-perception, "but listening to the imagery in the theories" (Padel 1992: 43).

With these propaedeutic considerations guiding us, we concentrated on two situations in which "the gene" surfaces in a conversation: on the one hand, the answers given when a concrete person is invited to voice his or her ideas about the term, its meaning, and its interpretation; and, on the other, the educational instruction about genes and their workings that genetic counselors impart to their clients. In one part of the project, we conducted interviews to elicit people's narratives about "genes," keeping in mind Jeannette Edwards's insistence on the "need for more sophisticated ways of hearing what [members of] 'the public' say about genetics" (Edwards 2002: 317). The interviewer was skilled in attentive listening and in carefully allowing the interviewee to articulate the ideas, notions, and experiences that the term evokes for her. Through these conversations we collected the oral material necessary to allow us to grasp what "genes" symbolically "say," and what they reflexively tell, command, and instill in people about who they are. In the second part of the research, we analyzed genetic counseling sessions in order to investigate what is said in the course of an expert's oral instruction. The conversation with an educator who has specialized in interpreting chromosome charts and biostatistics is supposed to enable the client to make a so-called autonomous decision about genetic tests. The counselor determines the client's risk profile by searching her medical history and family tree for potential genetic risks. From the risk profile, the array of test options is derived and the interventions' health risks, potential results, and possible actions to take are discussed. Thus, the geneticist speaks to a client and explains to the listening layperson in ordinary language the significance of genes for her health and for the decision she is asked to make. By assuming that the counselor's instructions help her to make an informed choice, the client accepts that the explanations about DNA structure and genetic risk assessment are of some importance to herself. What does the expert for biostatistics and genetic prognostications "say," intimate, or allude to in interactions with a concrete person?

We will first comment on the surprisingly incarnate and concrete semantics voiced in the gene talk of some interviews in a southern German village. Then we will discuss the symbolic fallout of professional education in genetics, namely, when genetic counselors address their clients as gene carriers and ascribe to them the need for risk awareness and self-management. The synthesis of both sections will allow us to draw first conclusions on the social symbolic function of gene talk.

THE "GENE IN HEUDORF"

In the course of one year (from the spring of 2003 through the spring of 2004), we talked to two dozen people in a southern German village, which we will call "Heudorf." The name is fictitious, yet the place with its 2,000 inhabitants is very real. We chose Heudorf as the location for our investigation for a variety of reasons: While located not far from a university town that contains a number of first-rate molecular biology institutes, the village itself remains even today a rather parochial, rustic place. The composition of the village population bridges different worlds and eras: It ranges from women taking pride in their lush, carefully tended gardens, which fill with calendula and phlox in the summer, to university administrators who spend their workdays gazing at computer screens.

Why fix an inquiry into "the gene" on two dozen people who live in such a place, most having little else in common? We deliberately abstained from talking to members of interest groups tied to science or politics, or groups of people who had become acquainted with genetics by being patients, and who had thus been formally introduced to key words prevalent in human genetics. By eliciting gene talk from people in one place, in one village, we hoped to ground genes (which by their very nature are a-topical) in the circumscribed horizon of a local topos and in the personal experiences and outlooks of these local people. The inhabitants of the village came from backgrounds varied enough to bring to the fore a variety of ideas on "genes" and genetics, as we spoke with people coming from the core of the old village—farmwomen and local craftspeople—and newcomers who had recently moved to Heudorf, including a Lutheran minister and a teacher. We began our investigation with a number of simple questions, and conducted the interviews accordingly: What expressive characteristics emerged in the range of responses? When do "genes" enter into personal deliberations? From what does the speaker derive his or her knowledge? What degree of assuredness or certainty did a speaker's mode of talking express about "genes"? And, finally, which figures of speech crop up with the greatest frequency? The interviews were prepared and conducted in such a way as to gain answers that would be personal, experiential, and as "real" as possible to the speaker. Our method of conducting the interviews draws from Pierre Bourdieu and Jean-Claude Kaufmann, both of whom have stressed the importance of listening to the speaker and of willingly engaging in a sympathetic, personal, and genuinely interested conversation.[3] We transcribed this material and scrutinized it along three discrete avenues: What do people say? What do "genes" "say" to people? And what does this gene talk tell the researcher about contemporary self-perception?

The first result was that an astounding variety of modes, inflections, and styles of speaking emerged. Elfriede, an old farmwoman, grumbled at these "inheritance things" (Vererbungsdinger), as she called them; and Marie-Sophie, the local hairdresser, talked about her aunt's, grandmother's, and uncle's suffering from all kinds of swellings and tumors, and related these to "genes." The teacher of physics and mathematics in the village primary school pontificated about "genes" as the origin of all "life on earth," while a philosophy professor who was unable to give a definition of DNA took "genes" to be the ultimate answer to questions already pondered by Aristotle, such as "What makes a human being?" The Lutheran minister told the interviewer that "God, yes, God the Creator, was the One who had made the genes," while by contrast, the conductor of the local brass orchestra and owner of a small printing press expressed strong reservations about the sense of talking about "genes" at all, because, as he said, "genes" are "alien" to Heudorf. And we arranged an interview with the woman who sells bread and pretzels in the local bakery because one morning we found her discussing the length of a chromosome string with a client over the counter, demonstrating it with her finger. We also spoke with others: the midwife, the woman working in the kindergarten, the apothecary, university students, and pupils from the village school. The register of responses we collected covered an immense range of concepts and ideas about "genes," and the tone, stance, and mode of speaking about them varied a great deal as well. Yet in listening to the material, certain common features of the "pop gene" began to puzzle us.

We will explore and illustrate one such characteristic here that has to do with the presumed fleshiness of the referent of the word: its puzzling ability to stand simultaneously for one's inherited bodily characteristics and for the determinative force, the inner actor that is supposed to be their cause. Our attention was drawn to this coexistence of "genes," which stand in for the familial past and the whole person as she is in the present, and as an invisible agent that might exercise a determinative force in the future. As our analysis of genetic counseling will show, it is exactly this ambiguity of the gene that ties risk prediction to bodily substance, merging two heterogeneous spheres: the statistical with the individual, the calculable with the unique and personal. To illustrate this ambiguity of genes in popular parlance, we will draw on the interviews of two women, the hairdresser Marie-Sophie and Petra, the woman in the bakery.

In a great number of other interviews as well, we found that the term *gene* was immediately and explicitly associated with something given that is the whole individual person. "Genes" in these accounts refer to incarnate semantics, to flesh and blood that can be felt, can be touched and seen. At the same time the speakers also attributed characteristics to "genes" that belong to a heterogeneous register or realm or sphere, one populated with genes that exercise a governing or determining influence over the person's makeup and her future. The semantic contours of these accounts also include elaborate stories about "manipulation," fantasies about cloned human beings and the creation of "catalogue-order babies," as well as fictional scenarios of ears or lungs or hearts grown in lab cultures. Thus we began to puzzle about these shifts in the semantic contours of the term from a synonym for somebody tangible, somatic, present—that is, flesh and blood—to some invisible, powerful, determining agent. We argue that it is by translation or transference from the flesh, per analogiam carnis, that the word *gene* can symbolically function as a vehicle for giving bodily substance to highly abstract notions. This translocation from the realm of the real or experiential to a sphere of the conjectured happens without a break, without a disruption, and without the speaker's awareness of the disparity inherent in the referent under discussion. Because "genes" in the first place are related to the whole person, past and present, the apperception of the whole person gives substance to fictional entities. Because of this echo in somatics, the abstract speculations in the genetic counseling sessions can appear as personally meaningful statements.

INCARNATE SEMANTICS: PASTS INCARNATE

In many of our interviewees' responses, we found a surprising eloquence and assuredness of people talking about their "genes." Most of our Heudorf respondents quickly began describing the word *gene* with the German term *Erbanlagen,* inherited traits, and they take it for granted that their very being can be explained with reference to this somatic inheritance. *Erbanlagen* is an old German compound. The word field of *Anlage* in colloquial German embraces a wide range of features of a person, among others character, being, trait, nature, disposition, personality, temper, or emotional life (Wahrig 1986: "Anlage," 168). The word names something constitutive of the person, and something that he or she interprets as inherited from his or her ancestors.

The saleswoman in the bakery ponders the fact that she physically resembles her grandmother, and she attributes these to *Erbanlagen* or "genes" bequeathed to her, saying,

Inheritance: that is—isn't it—like leaving me a house, you get it as a
present. And inheriting for me, as the saying goes, for me that is that
you have gotten it, you got it as a gift from him. But that was not a gift
in the outward sense, as if I handed over a parcel and said, I give you
that clock and your son will inherit this from you, but these are inner
things, you know, these are traits that we cannot influence.

In this sense of their "nature" that is given, genes are embedded in the
familial past and the somatic present. People vividly tell stories about characteristic personal features or striking traits, like the blue eyes of a person
or the curly hair of another or the blondness of a third, which are somehow,
colloquially, related to "genes"; and they evoke characteristic habits: the
way one looks, the quickness of one's intelligence, one's typical, habitual
gestures, or crotchets—how one holds a coffee cup, how one laughs.

The saleswoman in the bakery reports that her sister inherited an "Ital-
ian temperament" from her father, and the hairdresser speaks about her
nail-biting habit: "I think, yes, many habits and ways you move are simply
from genes...and I think you've got it inside you, as when you bite your
nails." Genes are thus in some sense both associated with the "nature"
with which one was endowed at birth and with second nature, the habits
one developed while growing up. The gene here is a term which points
toward the being in the now which one became through birth and after.
Inherited traits, *Anlage*, and Being are inseparable; there is no distinguish-
able difference between something as a cause and an effect or result. The
gene as *Erbanlage* is equivalent to that some-"body" one was endowed
with by being a son, a daughter, a grandson, and so forth, and the endowment manifests itself in the present. Gene stands in for origin, birth, and
something indisputable, for one's very being is the result of this endowment
through one's kinship ties. *Erbanlagen* is, as the hairdresser says, "what
you got in the cradle".

Marie-Sophie, the hairdresser, tells us the following:

Marie-Sophie: I think, certain features—those simply come from birth—or
from the very beginning. That's what it is. That's in the genes,
certain things—the proverbs say so. "That is in the genes." My
mother says so quite often. Me too. And I, I do think that's true.
Interviewer: Can you tell me what your mother meant when she said so?
Marie-Sophie: Yes, that this is as it is. It's given, it's predestined. That
the child has the same spleen or the same stubbornness, or
just the same habits that I have, or is just the way I was when I
was a child. That our [daughter] Sophie is such a troublemaker
[*Lumpenmensch*]. She gets into any mischief. I was just the same
in her age. First a nice baby, and then—oh dear. And my mother
used to say, "That's in her genes, you were the same. You have
given that to her." And my husband says, he says quite often,

"That's a gene that comes from me. [But] when [the children] are as cool as cucumbers and sit obediently still, very patient, then he says... "Oh, they have gotten something from me. That was one of my genes."

These proverbial "genes" that our interviewees take for granted refer to personal somatics, and they are identified in unmistakable habits and tastes. The semantic contours of the term are not far distant from those synonymous with the flesh that one is. These "genes" are rooted in the past, they bind the speaker to characteristics of his or her forebears, and for this reason they can be told in narratives, in familiar stories and anecdotes. Most people speak about their *Erbanlagen* with great confidence and conviction, and the sentences are punctuated with recurrent adverbial phrases, such as "certainly," "given," and "destined"—which express the perceptual mode of something unconditionally factual and indisputable. The "real mode" (modus realis) of these genes is also expressed in certain verbs that link genes to the past tense, that is, they are synonymous with a trait that one "received," that "was given." These genes, as the medical assistant who spoke to us affirms, colloquially substitute older, traditional expressions: "Like, this I got from my father, or my mother." Genes do not "become," but—as a synonym for the shared substance in kinship—they have been transmitted as flesh and blood, and "they are as they are."

A STABLE, FAMILIAL, SOMATIC ENDOWMENT FROM THE PAST INTO THE FUTURE

This perception of an incarnate endowment that was handed down in the flesh of the ancestors in some sense also reaches into the future. People are careful to make a distinction between this realm of something given and immutable—to which "genes" as synonym of flesh belong—and those spheres in life that can be influenced and changed by deliberate action. This is evident when the saleswoman in the bakery comments on the contrast between her familial—genetic—endowment and those actions and undertakings she can influence herself, or between "what is in the make-up and what can be made" (Edwards 2000). The saleswoman states,

If I eat as usual, I stay the same, but I can eat so that I lose weight. When I can influence things in my body with my mind or willfully, this is not a gene. I cannot do something about my size. I cannot change my eye color. Those are genes, but getting fat, or ruining your body by not washing yourself anymore, until I begin to stink like a goat or stop cutting my finger-nails, or simply mess around, that is no gene.

Because the semantic contours of the term embrace the flesh and blood one is, and because this is rooted in the factuality of the familial past, our respondents also voice certain expectations about the future. When the hairdresser talks about herself and her future, she refers to the same realm of factuality or inevitability:

> And everything that has been transmitted, I think, fits into the category of gene.... Many things are certainly predestined. There is a nice proverb—"I hope that you did not pass that on to me, so that I will turn out like him"...as cynical, or like my grandma was, or like that. My mother says so quite often, "I hope your father won't become like your grandma. He has many of her features, don't you think?"

The hairdresser is convinced that she will get varicose veins in the future because her mother suffered from them, and the woman in the bakery knows that later she will be plagued by headaches, just as her mother was. There is no room for the *modus irrealis* of unimaginable "maybe's" which we will later observe in the genetic counseling session. The future seems to be determined by what one already knows from experiences and by what one has observed in daily life. One's future physical destiny will be like the embodied familiar past.

In this register of Heudorf gene talk, the term *gene* is made synonymous with somatics and with "biology" in the old sense of that word, that is, one's curriculum vitae as embodied person. The word makes sense as proverbial wisdom and is embedded in experience, and the resulting knowledge belongs to the realm of those things that are certain to the speaker. Proverbs offer the condensed expression of many generations, and in this sense, as Mathilde Hain, a social anthropologist, observed, they form the concluding sentence of a chain of experiences (Hain 1951: 51).[4] Both our speakers found the validity of their reflections on "genes" on an authority: either a general "one says so" or through recourse to family members, as when the hairdresser insisted, "That's in the genes. My mother says so quite often." The proverbial expression "quotes an authority within which the certainties of a group have become the certainties of the person" (Hain 1951: 70). The word gene in this sense has nothing "genetic" about it. It is entirely incorporated into the colloquial idioms of kinship and heritage in which the speaker gives meaning to her existence.

DISTINCT, INVISIBLE, DETERMINING "GENES FOR"

In the course of the interviews, we tried to explore if and in what sense the interviewee would recognize a difference between *Erbanlagen* (hereditary factors) and "genes." "No," a single mother in the village reflects, "No, for me there is no difference—maybe there is a tiny difference, but I don't know of any." Yet the colloquial identification of *Erbanlagen* and flesh often takes on a different meaning because the word *gene* is understood to refer to something distinct, something internal and isolable, some biological "cause" or agent. The central verb changes in the same interview from being to having: These genetic *Erbanlagen* refer to something that the speaker "has," like an inner mark or essential factor. The term here reaches out to name a material entity that has the power to "make" or "determine" something. Within this frame, genes become synonymous to an underlying, invisible, and determinative cause for development. "Yes, there are genes," a home economics teacher says; "*Erbanlagen*, which are basic. Like, I need the genes, you know? Or cells that make my organs and my limbs and my hair." Within one interview, the two concepts may well coexist, yet the understanding of "genes" as a causative agent becomes more prevalent when the speaker has had a university education.

None of the interviewees, the local physician and the university students included, had the scientific terminology at hand to "correctly" define the gene, and there was an astounding range of ideas about the whereabouts of those "genes." Speakers assume them in the brain, in the blood, in particular cells all over the body, and the sentences in which they make an effort to come up with a definition are punctuated with signs of uncertainty. The whereabouts of these genes as invisible agents are a puzzle, but there is one definite characteristic about those hidden interior agents: Whatever is labeled with the word does have a determining power. The noun refers to a causative agency. Within this frame, the gene has the character of a command, of something apodictic, of some interior prescription. People talk about something being "genetically prescribed" or "determined in the cell division." The location, shape, and materiality of the referent of the term are definitely all over the map, but when people hypostatize "genes" as some distinct and isolable "thing," they attribute to this thing an active and determining power or capacity.

The hairdresser talks at length about homosexuality, which she thinks is imparted through birth:

> Yes, there simply are certain things that we have in our inheritance or that are genetically conditioned. That is simply so. As I've said a hundred times, being gay or lesbian is genetically determined. When the cells...divide after the third or fourth day, then at that moment, the heritage [Erbgut] or the genetic stuff... will be created.... Then it is determined whether a person is gay or lesbian.... It's just genetically determined, that someone is gay or lesbian. I am absolutely convinced that is how it is.

In clarifying the ways in which people spoke about these determining "genes for," it became clear to us that the power people attribute to them is, in a sense, tautological: These genes "make" what they are made to make.

Genes here are "genes for," and their potent power to make what they are made to affect is expressed in metaphors such as "building blocks" that underscore this character of the "gene" as a foundational cause of human existence. At this point, many interviewees begin to talk at length about "manipulation" or "cloning" or the future eradication of "deadly inherited diseases." For the argument we develop here, it is not this fantasy that is important, but the underlying idea that there are interior agents "for" something. "Genes" fuse with the conditions of which they are supposed to be the cause. This becomes clear when people muse about the fantastic possibilities that future research about "genes" will open up. Prevalent in this register of Heudorf gene talk is a figure of speech that takes the gene as a distinct building block for something, much as the apothecary says:

> If, for example, one would be able to define the gene for cancer, and could say: "Oh, man, we isolated that, now we know it's there and there, and now we can attack it by giving some drug...."—that would be a marvelous thing.

GENE DEFECT—DEFECTIVE GENES

The idea of genes as the cause of something that is already incorporated within them is most clearly expressed in those passages in our interviews that mention a neologism that has been spreading in ordinary German prose: "defective genes" or "gene defect." "Gene defect" is a syntagma, a compound that shifts the contours of the semantic field and locates "genes" within the realm of bad luck or unfortunate destiny.

This neologism has moved into ordinary speech in less than a decade. While the term gene had not yet appeared in the 1986 edition of *Wahrig's Deutsches Wörterbuch*, a German dictionary, the terms *defective gene* and *gene defects* gained currency as a vernacular rendering of "genetic mutation" during the 1990s. In our interviews the term is not infrequently mentioned, and it shows itself to be a newcomer with a strong connotative power. The term gene defect again implies that genes have real substance, as, logically, something must be there in order for it to be defective. As a compound, the word connects a tangible experiential property—brokenness, wrongness, defectiveness—with "genes" and thus imparts definite material substance to the term. Motors, cars, and televisions can be broken or can be defective. The interviewees draw from heterogeneous realms; they dress up the term, which alludes to something invisible, with the concrete properties that normally belong to the character attributed to the gene. The term *gene defect* is a lay reference to what is more strictly called the "genotype," even though this word does not appear in the Heudorf interviews. But, characteristically, this way of referring to the genotype objectifies it in the definite shape of some "thing" that has the capacity to be broken or wrong.

The nurse in the kindergarten declares,

A defect is something that does not run properly, I don't know, this is what the encyclopedia says, or so, if something is defective, that means it's broken or needs to be fixed, along these lines.

In her explanation, the nurse testifies to the inevitable concretization of "genes" when they are linked to the semantic field of mistake or wrongness: Concrete images taken from mechanics abound, and so the referent of the word takes on the semblance of a real "something" with an astounding range of properties that the "defectiveness" brings with it: crooked, askew, uneven, curved, odd, not straight, wrong, ill-fitting,—or "something is missing". This is how the hairdresser defines the compound:

Gene defect? To say this in a simple way, I think, each human being does have a certain number of genes in the body. There are enumerations, as far as I know. I have heard about it, but I can't explain it further. But, I do think, each gene probably must have a certain form, or a certain task in the body. And if this is going the wrong way.... Maybe all these genes should be in one row, as you see with the molecules...when they all stand in one row. When they all stand next to each other... the chain is whole. And maybe it is like that with a gene defect...they should stand one after the other, but they do not. They are out of place [*versetzt*] or one is missing. This is how I do imagine it.

Several times in the interview, she comes up with images she had learned in chemistry classes when being trained as a hairdresser, and the image of molecules chained in a row or maybe that of chromosomes lined up, one next to the other, fit into her idea of defective genes. Again we find the figure of speech that identifies cause and effect as one and the same. There are a number of verbs that show how people invest the "defective genes" with the simple unilinear capacity to do something, in this case to do the wrong things. We quote from the verbs used: "It does not function as it should ordinarily," "it runs wrong," "it's not working the right way," "it's producing the wrong things," "it's going wrong," and "it's failing."

Gene defect is a term that compounds a notion of "genes for"; genes as a determining cause, with the apparent effect of that supposed cause. Genes here are not imagined as a factor in the development of a condition, but rather as a something shaped in the likeness of the crookedness that will appear or is already apparent in the person. The nurse coins an apt term for this when she speaks of the "crooked-growth genes" (Krummwachs-Gen). In one compound, she invests the imagined shape of the underlying determining cause with traits she has seen with her own eyes—something or someone "crooked." The human being then is just a "receptacle" within which genes to do their appointed job (Finkler 2000: 20). The shape of this idea is not to be confused with the notion of risk in genetic counseling. "Risk" is a purely statistical concept, whereas a wrong or defective gene is imagined analogous to the very condition of the person it is supposed to have made.[5]

"THE GENE" AS LATENT MENACE

Finally, striking are the passages in the narratives of Petra, the woman working in the bakery, when she comes up with images of "genes" that belong to another realm: the realm of chance when "genes" act unpredictably. In the following quote, Petra reifies the gene in the image of Pandora's box, an image embodying a latent threat. When she is asked if she would do the same as those American women she had read and talked about who had their breasts removed after a "positive" predictive test result for breast cancer, she says,

> No…but I would regularly go to the doctor. Because the gene, the gene might not necessarily break out in me. It can be like a capsule, you know, just like AIDS. That you have AIDS, but it is not yet real. It is like a sealed box. I had my kidney stones over years and the doctor said, "If they do not move, then you might get old with your kidney stones. But mind you, if one starts to move!" That's it. Sometimes I imagine genes like a capsule. If, for example, they find out that you have this and that gene. Is it 100 percent sure that this will happen? Has it opened already, the gene? In all likelihood it is like a capsule. And because of some influence…I do not know what, the thing breaks open, and only then, it comes.

The image of a sealed capsule that might or might not "open" strikingly reifies a very new meaning of the word. Our interviewee speaks of a menacing interior latency which threatens a catastrophic outbreak. It is probably no accident that this image came up in Petra's narrative since she had undergone prenatal genetic counseling. There, she learned about hidden mutations, risk distributions, and their portents for her coming child. As the other interviews show, the concept of genetic susceptibility which is so strikingly pictured in the "capsule" has not gained wide currency in Heudorf. It clashes with their register of imagined genes. The strong, definitive, and determining chain of somatic endowment that links them to the past, to their kin and their belief in mechanical causation, leaves little room for chance or multifactorial interrelated probabilities. The concept of a "latency"—as concretized in the "capsule"—that is physically present and at the same time incorporates a "maybe" that might or might not show in the future, will be the basic characteristic of the gene in genetic counseling. But it still seems to be alien to the Heudorf mental and physical cosmos.

The characteristics of the "gene" in the Heudorf narratives should be kept in mind when we now look at the information about "genes" that a genetic counselor imparts to a client. In Heudorf, the word refers to something eminently factual, personal, sensual, and somatic, and also to an invisible powerful determining agent, a something that can be wrong or broken. In any case, the referent of the term seems plausible to the speaker because it points to his or her somatic endowment. In light of the genetic counseling sessions, we will see how the proverbial "I and my genes" is the precondition for the client's seeing rhyme and reason in the geneticist's instruction about "your genetic risks." It is by analogy with the flesh that the term *gene* gives bodily substance to highly abstract notions such as "risk" and "probability." In this way, the social symbolic function of parlance about "genes" becomes visible: We will see how the counselor's references to "genes" literally implant population statistics, probabilistic reasoning, and the need for self-management in the corporeal makeup of the person addressed as a gene carrier.

GENETIC COUNSELING AS A CALL
FOR SELF-MANAGEMENT

Genetic counseling is a professional service that aims to activate people into becoming responsible consumers of genetic tests, statistical predictions, and so-called preventive measures. As we will see, the genetic counselors' "pop gene," from which they derive risk predictions, differs fundamentally from the embodied, carnal narratives in Heudorf. Genetic counselors speculate about the possibility that a client—or a client's offspring—will contract certain diseases in the future. All they can specify is what might happen and place the "might" into a statistical frame. Based on the family history and, if available, genetic test results, geneticists support this fortune telling with probability figures calculated on the basis of statistical tables and formulas. In prenatal genetic counseling, the geneticist assigns every client a so-called basic risk of 5 percent that something is wrong with the child and makes sure that she becomes aware of everything that could happen. Then the counselor ascribes to the pregnant woman her "personal risk" (e.g., 1:435 or 1:100) to expect a child with Down's syndrome.[6] In genetic counseling around cancer, the geneticist assigns the client a "genetic risk" for breast or colon cancer. As the counselors' information suggests, all these calculations and predictions are based on "genes," that is, the stuff—as the interviews in Heudorf have shown—which is considered to make and have made the embodied person, the being-as-it-is. Thus, the calculated probabilities seem to identify a threat already lurking inside the body.

Our analysis of the social symbolic function of professional education on genes and genetic risks is based on eighteen genetic counseling sessions which the geneticist in our team has observed and tape-recorded in three different genetic counseling centers in Germany. In a previous study, she examined the paradoxes of "taught self-determination" (Samerski 2003). For that, she listened to thirty genetic counseling sessions and chose thirteen of them for detailed analysis. For our project on the pop gene, we transcribed fourteen of the remaining recordings, and observed and tape-recorded four more counseling sessions at a cancer genetics clinic.

For two reasons we chose this ritual as an instance for the study of the pop gene. First, geneticists talk to laypeople. They have to spell out their knowledge so that ordinary people can follow them. To do so, the expert has to find everyday words for concepts like chromosomal aberrations, DNA mutation, and probability model. Second, the aim of the lesson is not only to enlighten the clients but also to prepare them for a decision they are urged to make. Today, the explicit goal of such counseling is the client's choice on the basis of genetic and statistical constructs. It converted from hereditary prognostications and eugenic prevention into a service industry selling information, knowledge, and reassurance as necessary raw materials for informed decision about test options. Thus, facing the counselors' explanations, clients rightly expect them to say something concrete and tangible about them. They inevitably ask themselves: What does all this say about me? What does all this mean to me? Therefore, genetic counseling is a privileged instance to investigate how the pop gene reinterprets self-understanding and deliberation.

In five of the eighteen counseling sessions analyzed for our project, a geneticist—here a woman—informed her clients about the genetic basis and statistical distribution of a certain type of cancer. Those seeking counseling had lost sisters, a father, or an aunt to colon or breast cancer and feared they might share the same fate. After the counseling session, clients had not learned anything about themselves or their future well-being, nor were they more familiar with scientific thinking. But they had learned something else: They had been taught that genes matter, and that these genes can pose a serious threat to their health and to their future. And this belief in the existence and power of genes paves the way for a fundamental transformation of the client's self-understanding. Thinking of herself as a gene carrier, she is prepared to take statistical calculations and probability curves as meaningful statements about herself and her family. Since the counseling ritual and the expert's colloquial formulations cause her to believe that the information is about her, the one who is sitting there, she is ready to confuse the attribution of a risk profile with a doctor's diagnosis. Thus, professional enlightenment about genes and genetic risks teaches clients to see themselves from the point of view of an insurance broker or of a health economist. It demands from them to manage themselves as abstract risk profiles.

CORRELATION AS CAUSE

The following sequences taken from a session on breast cancer demonstrate how statistical speculations gel into a diagnosis, a personal threat which then hangs over the client's present-day life like a Damoclean sword. The geneticist explained to the worried woman that there were so-called high-risk families that carry a genetic program for breast cancer. A test could clarify whether she had also inherited this program. A "minimal change"[7] in DNA is supposedly responsible for this cruel fate, explained the counselor. In this logic, suffering and death are reduced to the ultimate event in an invisible chain of defects and malfunctions. The client, in her mid-forties, seemed to be healthy, yet the catastrophe could have already begun in her body. Her body might not be functioning well on the molecular level, as the counselor informed her:

Counselor: And there is this so-called protein molecule whose function has changed or is defective compared to its normal function in the body. And this is what ultimately leads this carrier toward cancer.

A few sentences later, however, the counselor conceded that this biochemical change was not the cause of breast cancer. She states clearly that even with a positive test result, it would still be a matter of speculation whether the woman facing her would contract breast cancer:

Counselor: So if a change in BRCA 1 or 2 is carried…
Client: Yes…
Counselor:…a woman carrying this change has, statistically seen—which says nothing at all about individuals—a lifelong risk of about 80–85 percent of getting breast cancer.

Leaving aside the question of the accuracy of those numbers,[8] they mean that one fifth of those diagnosed as BRCA gene carriers do not get breast cancer. And no one can explain why some get it and others do not. Thus the mutation does not have any causal relation to the disease, but is merely a trait that places a person in a risk group that contracts breast cancer more often than average. The genetic defect is a shorthand for a probabilistic relationship between genotype and phenotype.[9] Nevertheless, as the counselor clarified in her next sentence, she perceived the number as alarming and felt the need to warn her client:

Counselor: Now these are very high numbers…
Client: Hmm.
Counselor:…which means you need to be careful. And that's why we recommend [short pause] frequent screening for early detection.

A statistical calculation has become a bodily menace. One's own body has been turned into the major threat to one's own health. By conjuring up an alarming threat on the grounds of risk figures, the counselor asks her client to go out of her mind and body. She is supposed to swing back and forth on a statistically constructed temporal axis that means to leave the present and place herself in a probabilistically precalculated future. In one of these future possibilities, she has breast cancer. Carrying the knowledge of what might—perhaps—happen, she is to return to the present and make it her perspective for thinking, feeling, and acting today. She is then to do everything in her power to make sure this possible event, that is, breast cancer, does not occur—an event that no one can really determine will occur or not. She must act, today, to ward off phantoms of the future.

The woman who had appeared at this counseling session has not yet received any genetic test results. But because she comes from a family in which breast cancer has occurred at an early age and on both sides, she is considered to be a so-called high-risk person—just to be on the safe side, the counselor emphasizes, since they don't want to lull her into a false sense of security. A genetic test would confirm this status, or yield no results and thus do nothing to change this risk classification, or reduce her statistical risk of getting breast cancer. A negative genetic test would give her a different classification, dropping her risk down to the average:

Counselor:...which basically could then put your risk of getting breast cancer, from a statistical perspective, down to the average risk.

She might still get breast cancer, even without the BRCA gene. But now if she becomes ill, without the feared gene, her breast cancer would be classified differently: it would be considered "nonhereditary." The counselor explains to her client, "Say your cousin tested positive and you didn't, and you still get breast cancer, they'd then say it wasn't hereditary."

GENES AS STOREHOUSES FOR POSSIBILITIES

"Genes," however, open up more than one frightening possibility. They broaden the spectrum of fearsome potentialities, the horizon of things that might happen. With the amount of sequence information on the human genome growing, statisticians use the flood of data to calculate correlations between DNA and clinical symptoms. These probabilities express nothing but abstract frequencies. In the consulting room, however, these frequencies are pinned on clients as "genetic risks." In a session where the client is worried because several of her relatives were suffering of colon cancer, the counselor links the potential genetic defect to a host of other future possibilities no less alarming than the first.

Counselor: And then there are other types of cancer found in these families. And they can include, uh...an increased occurrence of stomach cancer. [Client rolls her eyes.]... Um, [pause] then um, [short
pause] there is ovarian cancer [client leans forward, her eyes wide
with concern] that can occur more frequently, that is, it is not
rare, so it is very important for you to undergo gynecological
screening.... No? Then um, there is also a more frequent occurrence of cancer in the efferent urinary tract [client furrows her
forehead and raises her eyebrows].

The "gene" here is a kind of storehouse of different possibilities that
might occur in the future and with which the woman must reckon. The
counselor recommends preventive measures for each of these possibilities.
The woman who originally was afraid of getting colon cancer must now
undergo ultrasound tests and cytological investigations every year to make
sure that she does not also have cervical cancer, stomach cancer, or ure-
thral cancer.

THE PERSON AS A MANAGEABLE CONSTRUCT

The genetic counselors' information on gene mutations and cancer risks did
not add an iota to her client's knowledge about herself and her future. With
or without gene testing, nobody can know if the woman sitting at the counselor's table will get cancer or not. The genetic counselor could only speculate on what might happen; her statements were interlaced with expressions
such as "if ...then," "it could," "it would," or a general "there are." In contrast to Heudorf, where the people's narratives express the perceptual mode
of something factual and indisputable, the genetic counselor mainly speaks
in the hypothetical subjunctive, the modus potentialis. Thereby, he creates
a new kind of anxiety, namely, risk anxiety: "It is exactly these uncertainties that enable marketeers to exploit fears: fears of birth defects, 'problem'
pregnancy and disease. Speculation almost unnoticeably shades into prediction, as genetic screening becomes a 'probability statement about future
risk'" (van Dijck 1998: 98). But the power and symbolic efficacy of genetic
fortune telling can only be understood when both sides of the pop gene, the
fictitious and the embodied, are taken into consideration. It is the unreality,
the speculative nature of the expert's gene talk on the one hand, and the
concrete, bodily meaning of genes in everyday parlance on the other hand,
that make genetic predictions so powerful.

The geneticist's expertise is based on the statistical homogenization
of individuals and the probabilistic characteristics of fictive cohorts. The
fact that she addresses her client personally in colloquial language merely
obscures the gulf between the person before her and the data record from

which her statements derive. Thus, the counselor's colloquial explanations of highly abstract, statistical relations lead to an entirely new form of inconsistency in conversations. Listening to a geneticist across the table, the client feels addressed while hearing about a potential gene defects and "her individual risk." The referent of these technical terms and the addressee of the information, however, are incompatible. A "risk" and a "gene for" refer to the frequency of occurrences in statistical populations and never to the "I" or "you" in a colloquial statement. By merging personal reference and statistics, the client is asked to see herself as a construct whose being-as-it-is is a patchwork of characteristics from statistical classes. But this far-reaching remodeling of the person as a calculable "gene carrier" is not an avoidable side effect of the counseling session, but its implicit goal. Only when the client sees herself as a gene carrier and risk profile does she adapt herself and become physically compatible with the logic of cost-benefit analyses and economically oriented decision making. The goal of genetic counseling is to teach the client a new form of responsibility, that is, managerial decision making in the shadow of risk. This requires replacing the unique and personal "I" and "you" with statistical constructs, with risk profiles. By convincing clients that the—probable—fates precalculated and assigned to them by experts are already preprogrammed in their bodies, namely, in their genes, counselors are asking them to turn themselves into the very resource required for risk-guided management of populations.

CONCLUSION

Elizabeth Shea (2001) has drawn attention to the fact that in contemporary cultural usage, "genes" are often used like traditional commonsense nouns in which they take on the same status as pots and pans, tables or chairs. She traces the usage of the term in the history of biology, where for almost a century "gene" had the status of a conceptual tool, a word naming not a miniscule material entity but the hypothetical cause behind a visible effect, a trait, a feature which was attributed to this black-boxed underlying cause. This particular status of the term has given it a unique metonymic power so that simultaneously in the course of its history it could refer to some invisible material referent, some unit of heredity, or the developmental processes derived from the supposed referent's power to do or make something. "Even at their most literal genes are already caught in a helix of materiality and abstraction," she writes, and she explains the persuasiveness of genes in contemporary culture in this characteristic to accommodate a unique "material-abstract ambiguity" (Shea 2001: 508, 509). Shea posits that this has changed in the last decades:

> The metonymic function that has enabled the gene, throughout the twentieth century, to figure a sense of reality has become camouflaged

as the material realities of genes have been established by molecular genetics, endorsed by the human genome project, and celebrated in the popular press. (2001: 516)

But, as cutting-edge research in genetics has shown, the material reality of "genes" cannot be established (Beurton et al. 2000). In molecular biology, the hypothesis of "genes" as distinct determining building blocks of all life is an outdated paradigm; however, the willingness of the layperson to believe in a deterministic "gene for" has grown in inverse proportion to the demise of this concept in science. The rhetorical figure of the "gene" today performs a social function that goes beyond the mind-shaping power of a popular cultural icon. Outside of the boundaries of laboratory science and data processing, the word "gene" has attained an extraordinary property: In one breath, it refers to what is most concrete, personal, and intimate—the soma of the speaker or the addressed—while at the same time referring to statistical probabilities and risk profiles. In ordinary language, the "gene" encapsulates the potency to perform an alchemical transformation: The term merges soma with statistics. Inevitably—if this is noticed or not—gene talk transmutes the speaker's or listener's very flesh and blood into a something made out of "genes," and thus makes the embodied person equivalent to a "case" to which the logic of large numbers, statistical probabilities, and chance adheres.

By putting under scrutiny the key word, the lemma *gene*, and doing so in the domain of laypeople's understanding and at the moment of its crossing over from scientific discourse into everyday speech, we analyzed the latent functions of "gene" as a neologism. The gulf between heterogeneous modes of reasoning and disparate logics that the term bridges and coalesces became glaringly apparent: Cause and correlation, sensual awareness and probability calculations, the somatic "I" and risk profiles tend to be confounded. Other researchers observed the extreme but logical consequence of this implantation of a latent threat into one's own flesh. In interviews with women whose physicians have attributed an increased risk of cancer to them, one of the women would prefer to have everything cut out of her body that she does not really need in order to live, "because the tiniest bit can go wrong, and if that's not there, well, you can't have a problem with it" (Kavanagh & Broom 1998). Her sentence is an epitome for the power of the deictic somatic reference of a term that bespeaks the somatic "I" and "you" in the logic of their des-incarnation.

NOTES

1. Since her first exegesis of these early eighteenth-century medical protocols, Duden has again and again adopted the perspective of disciplined estrangement: looking at the present from the point of view of former sensual perceptions and vice versa; see also Duden (2002).

2. This statement of course is an oversimplification, yet we have often been astonished about the belief in the existence of "genes" among colleagues, which fosters an epistemic conundrum: how to take distance from the certainties that one perceives as embodied. In the course of our research, we found helpful the ethnographic work of Kaja Finkler (2000) and Jeannette Edwards (2000).

3. Bourdieu (1999) elaborates on his method in conducting interviews in a way that helps the interviewee bring forth ideas that had not previously emerged in the light of consciousness, and Jean-Claude Kaufmann has systematized this approach in Kaufmann (2004).

4. Hain has collected and analyzed the character of colloquial, proverbial language in a village 100 km north of Frankfurt am Main. Her work today is particularly illuminating because she recorded the talk of people in daily life before the great transformation of ways of talking under the influence of popularized sociological terminology occurred. Hain concluded that colloquial speech frames individual experience in a general relationship, and because it shapes this experience as generally valid, it invests what is being said with authority.

5. Mette Nordahl Svendsen (2004: 4ff.) describes this transformation of quantitative probabilities into supposed bodily substances; see the second part of our investigation, below.

6. On the meaning and function of "risk" in prenatal genetic counseling, see Samerski (2002).

7. All quotations are taken verbally from our transcripts.

8. For a critique of those numbers as too high because of a biased study design, see Begg (2002).

9. This 85 percent risk refers to a life expectancy of seventy-five years, and nobody knows whether the client will live to this age or will die at sixty-eight of a heart attack. However, statistical figures not only cannot be interpreted outside their original context; they also per se can say nothing about a concrete person—the counselor concedes this quite explicitly.

REFERENCES

Begg, Collin. 2002. On the use of familial aggregation in population-based case probands for calculating penetrance. *Journal of the National Cancer Institute* 94, no. 16: 1221–26.

Beurton, Peter; Hans-Jörg Rheinberger, and Raphael Falk, eds. 2000. *The concept of the gene in development and evolution: Historical and epistemological perspectives.* Cambridge: Cambridge University Press.

Bourdieu, Pierre. 1999. *The weight of the world: Social suffering in contemporary society.* Stanford, CA: Stanford University Press.

Duden, Barbara. 1991. *The woman beneath the skin: A doctor's patients in eighteenth-century Germany.* Cambridge, MA: Harvard University Press.

———. 2002. *Die Gene im Kopf, der Fötus im Bauch. Historisches zum Frauenkörper.* Hannover: Offizin Verlag.

Edwards, Jeannette. 2000. *Born and bred: Idioms of kinship and new reproductive technologies in England.* Oxford: Oxford University Press.

———. 2002. Taking "public understanding" seriously. *New Genetics and Society* 21, no. 3: 315–25.

Finkler, Kaja. 2000. *Experiencing the new genetics: Family and kinship on the medical frontier.* Philadelphia: University of Pennsylvania Press.

Hain, Mathilde. 1951. *Sprichwort und Volkssprache. Eine volkskundlich-soziologische Dorfuntersuchung.* Giessen: Schmitz.

Kaufmann, Jean-Claude. 2004. *L'entretien compréhensif.* Paris: Armand Colin.

Kavanagh, A. M., and D. H. Broom. 1998. Embodied risk: My body, myself? *Social Science and Medicine* 46:437–44.

Nordahl Svendsen, Mette. 2004. "The journey of the gene": Pasts conceptualized and futures imagined in cancer genetic counseling. Paper presented at 4S/EAAST, August 26–28, Paris.

Padel, Ruth. 1992. *In and out of the mind: Greek images of the tragic self.* Princeton, NJ: Princeton University Press.

Samerski, Silja. 2002. *Die verrechnete Hoffnung: Von der selbstbestimmten Entscheidung durch genetische Beratung.* Münster: Westfälisches Dampfboot.

———. 2003. Entmündigende Selbstbestimmung: Wie die genetische Beratung schwangere Frauen zu einer unmöglichen Entscheidung befähigt. In *Verkörperte Technik—Entkörperte Frau: Biopolitik und Geschlecht,* edited by Sigrid Graumann and Ingrid Schneider, 213–29. Frankfurt am Main: Campus Verlag.

———. 2005. Autonomy and therapy. *New Perspectives Quarterly* 22, no. 1: 71–77.

Shea, Elizabeth. 2001. The gene as rhetorical figure: "Nothing but a very applicable little word." *Science as Culture* 10, no. 4: 505–29.

van Dijck, José. 1998. *Imagenation: Popular images of genetics.* London: Macmillan.

Wahrig. 1986. *Deutsches Wörterbuch.* Gütersloh: Distribooks.

11 Genetics and its publics
Crafting genetic literacy and identity in the early twenty-first century

Karen-Sue Taussig

In April 2003 Francis Collins, director of the U.S. National Human Genome Research Institute, and his colleagues published a feature article in the journal *Nature* in which they articulated three major themes for the future of genomics—genomics to biology, genomics to health, and genomics to society (Collins et al. 2003). In conceptualizing the relationships among these themes, they describe—and provide a graphic image of—a three-story house. The caption under their image of this genomic abode—a three-story Frank Lloyd Wright-style house—states that "the future of genomics rests on the foundation of the Human Genome Project." Sitting first upon this foundation on the ground floor is their theme of "genomics to biology." They designate the second floor as "genomics to health," while the third floor, supported by all this science and medicine, they allot to the theme of genomics to society.[1]

This surely is an interesting image about which much could be said, and the anthropological literature has long pointed to houses as metaphors for social collectivities, particularly that modern form we know as the nation-state. But why do Francis Collins and his colleagues see these themes, organized as a house, as central to their vision of the future of genomics? However useful their image, their goal is to emphasize the Human Genome Project's new focus on translational research; that is, the translation of genomic knowledge into genomic interventions into human health that will benefit society by improving the health of individuals and of populations.

Collins et al. (2003) describe what they call "six cross-cutting elements" that they illustrate as pillars running through all the floors of their house. They designate these elements as resources; technology development; computational biology; training; ethical, legal, and social implications (ELSI); and education. I am particularly interested in what Collins and his colleagues describe as "resources," including the development of databases of "cohort populations for studies designed to identify genetic contributions to health ... including a 'healthy' cohort," and in their focus on what they describe as "education"—for them, in part, a population educated to know how to appropriately consume genetic knowledge and technologies.

Genome scientists have persistently promised that although there would be a "therapeutic lag," the funding of the Human Genome Project (HGP)—in the United States with $3 billion—would pay off in dramatic interventions into human health. They have promised that, however distant, the knowledge the project would produce would teach us fundamental things about biology that would translate into development of significant treatments for the widespread common conditions compromising human health. While the project itself has beat every deadline in terms of the production of knowledge, that knowledge has not yet led to the kinds of health interventions the project's promoters have always promised. One geneticist, for example, has quipped, "With regard to understanding the A's, T's, G's, and C's of genomic sequence, by and large, we are functional illiterates" (cited in Fox Keller 2000: 6). The idea of translational research has been so central to the project that the fact that these translations have not yet occurred is of increasing concern to geneticists. As one put it to me over a year ago, "[P]eople are starting to ask, 'What have you done for us lately?'"

For the past few years, I have been tracking the effort to develop genomic medicine in relation to the material demands of contemporary genetic knowledge production. I am interested in the ways contemporary desires for medical interventions into human life and health and for the material means of contemporary research in the life sciences—DNA, family histories, and medical records—now converge to bring new biosocial forms into being. As Eugene Chan, the founder and chairman of U.S. Genomics, put it in a 2002 article in the business section of the New York Times, "To truly understand genomics, you are going to need access to millions of genomes" (Riordan, 2002). It is, of course, exactly this realization that provides the theoretical underpinnings for the development of the Icelandic company DeCode Genetics, which has turned virtually every Icelandic citizen into a research subject (Fortun 2001; Rose 2001; Sigurdsson 2001; Specter 1999).

My research aims to understand this 'naturalcultural' production through investigating whether and how the practices emerging with new genetic knowledge engender new kinds of selves, persons, and citizens.[2] In my research I am arguing that we are in the midst of a profound worldview shift regarding genetic causality and responsibility for human health, engendering new biopolitical regimes and related social and embodied practices. I argue that the contemporary biopolitics being forged by desires for genomic medicine configures persons as biosocial citizens whose bare life is essential for the production of knowledge and control of the health of individuals and populations and whose ethical life is being crafted as demanding participation in the knowledge production process.[3] A number of social theorists of highly diverse theoretical orientations suggest that we are in a moment of major historical transformation in which developments in the life sciences play a significant role (e.g., Agamben 1995/1998; Fukuyama 2002; Habermas 2001; Rose, this volume). Here I offer a series of examples that illustrate these social processes in action. I do so in order to illustrate their diversity as well as to highlight the roles played by ordinary people in the production of scientific knowledge and its corresponding social forms. All of these examples come from the United States; they reflect and serve to produce and reproduce distinctive aspects of U.S. culture.

In those countries where genomics is culturally relevant and socially available, new genetic knowledge makes claims on transforming conceptualizations of health and illness, on how people imagine their relationships to each other, on human variation, and even on understandings of what it is to be human. Effecting the translation of genomic knowledge to genomic medicine would seem essential to achieving the "genomic era" genome scientists have promised. Efforts are now underway to develop an approach to medicine in which genes are seen to play a role in every aspect of human biology, including many widespread conditions such as heart disease, asthma, and cancer. In talking about this new knowledge and its potential application in molecular medicine, geneticists, physicians, and others make claims on its transformative powers, insisting that it will transform society as we have previously known it by, for example, likening its emergence to harnessing electricity. This is also a highly capitalized area of the contemporary market. Both large multinational pharmaceutical companies and individuals have invested enormous amounts of finance capital into a complex, multilayered, biotechnology industry that does everything from harvest and store DNA to carry out research focused on developing marketable knowledge or products. But the kind of transformations these various cultural and capital investments depend upon cannot just happen. New ways of thinking about the world do not simply seep into the collective unconscious. Nor do new social and embodied practices emerge from nowhere. These transformations can only be effected, first, if they have some basis in material reality and, second, if they are taught, learned, and experienced.

MINING DNA

If it is going to take millions of genomes to "truly understand genomics" and if we need a population educated in genetics so that they will properly participate in understanding and consuming genomic knowledge, what social processes are at work in attempting to make this "genomic era" a reality? Today a wide array of social activities are underway that aim to develop the kind of molecular medicine so clearly desired by some scientists, physicians, the biotechnology industry, and those living with compromising health conditions. The work aimed at making this genomic era a reality does involve millions of genomes, and, thus, it focuses, in part, on mining and contextualizing DNA and on educating people so that they will participate in genetic research. In other words, this work is about resources and education, major pillars supporting the genomic abode imagined by Francis Collins and his colleagues.

Gaining access to DNA for research purposes in a society such as the United States is a daunting proposition. The United States has a well-documented history of medical and scientific abuses; it also is organized around a legal system and ideological regimes based on individualism, individual rights, and privacy; it has no national health care system; and it has a maze of Internal Review Board (IRB) and informed consent processes that are widely recognized as unwieldy and inadequate. When it comes to the rare, obviously genetic conditions, gaining access to the material means of knowledge production is a relatively simple matter. Desperate families with sick children are far more concerned to enroll clinicians and researchers in their search for treatment than they are about just about anything else. As genetic activists Sharon and Patrick Terry pointed out to me, putting an informed consent form in front of a family with a genetic condition is "like throwing them a rope. Of course they're going to grab on." Recruiting the large number of participants required for research on the more widespread common conditions now viewed as having a genetic component is much more complicated. When it comes to research on common conditions, people appear far less willing to participate.

Contemporary efforts to gain access to DNA are quite diverse. Some stem from the desires of individuals and families bearing compromising genetic conditions to further research agendas that may lead to valuable treatments. Others originate with powerful medical institutions seeking to enroll a wide array of individuals in medical/scientific research. The various efforts I have observed each frame and inform genetic knowledge and practice in different ways. They also each construct complex and contested identities that variously enable or constrain the agency and voice of those people they seek to engage in genetic knowledge and practice. Exploring the range of ways researchers and others are attempting to develop the material basis of molecular medicine throws into relief the relationships among science, the state, patients, and others in the production of genetic literacy and identity in the twenty-first century.

FAMILIES

Along with geneticists, perhaps those who have the greatest concern to develop molecular medicine are those people organized as what are referred to as "patients' groups." These are the desperate families with sick children who testify before Congress and often serve as the legitimating figures for genetic knowledge production. Although their story is not typical, Sharon and Pat Terry's work as genetic activists offers a model of crafting genetic social relations. In 2000, Sharon Terry was a coauthor on two back-to-back articles in *Nature Genetics*, announcing the discovery of the gene for *pseudoxanthoma elasticum* (PXE) (Bergen et al. 2000; Le Saux et al. 2000), and Pat Terry joined Randy Scott—the founder and former CEO of Incyte, a major biotechnology company—and three others in securing $70 million in venture capital to establish Genomic Health, a new biotechnology firm.

Their story begins, however, several years earlier. Patrick Terry, a technical high school graduate with two years of study at a community college, was managing a construction company, and Sharon Terry, who has a master's degree in religious studies, was home-schooling their son and daughter when the children were diagnosed with PXE in 1994. Following their children's diagnosis, the Terrys beat a path to the University of Massachusetts medical school library, more than sixty kilometers from their home. There they copied over 400 articles on PXE and began educating themselves on the state of knowledge about the condition. Realizing how little was known about the condition, the Terrys resolved to facilitate research for the benefit of their children. They learned about a physician researching the condition and contacted him. Describing that encounter, Sharon Terry explains that the physician told them,

> "PXE's a rat-hole. Nobody cares. No one will ever care about this disease. I gave my life to it. You only have me." And we kept saying, "Well, we think we could interest other people if we could get enough people's blood samples."... You know, that sort of thing? And he kept saying, "No, you can't."... But...that same night he introduced us to a researcher [at Harvard]... a fellow who was working on PXE, looking for the gene.... So we said to the fellow, "We'll wash test tubes for you, just to accelerate your research. What do you want done?" This same group had taken our blood and tissue...the day after my kids were diagnosed without an informed consent from us. We didn't...know at the time that you're supposed to have one. We were...grateful that somebody wanted our blood.

The Terrys began volunteering in the laboratory of this Harvard researcher, frequently working through the middle of the night. At the same time, committed to enrolling additional researchers in order to speed up results and develop a treatment, the Terrys founded PXE International. One role of the organization was to bank patients' tissue, develop pedigrees, and maintain an international registry of affected individuals and families. These materials are just what geneticists seek in their effort to further develop genetic knowledge. A comprehensive tissue bank linked to medical records, family pedigrees, and so on provides a unique picture of what a specific condition actually looks like, thus facilitating researchers' ability to understand the complex pathways from gene to expression. The Terrys frame their mission this way:

What is it that researchers need to do their job? Blood, tissue, pedigrees, family studies. And how do we solve this problem?... We hold the key and the gold. We hold 900 blood samples, 200 pedigrees, and 1,400 affected individuals and they have to come to us for them. And we know that that is real power.

Thus, by maintaining control over the material means of scientific knowledge production, the Terrys and their organization are participating in and shaping the basic research process itself. At the same time, they are also shaping the researchers' understandings of what it means to live with this condition.

The Terrys' efforts led to rapid development of contemporary scientific capital—the development of new knowledge involving the discovery and naming of a new gene. At the same time, they protected the concerns of patients about privacy and control. In this case, people were willing to participate in research not only because they had a rare genetic condition (which they had always had) but also because they trusted the Terrys to maintain control over their materials, to protect their privacy, and to push for the interests of people with PXE.

In June 2000, the same week that President Bill Clinton, Francis Collins, and Craig Venter announced the completion of the rough draft of the human genome, PXE International held a celebratory dinner dance at Boston's Park Plaza Hotel, commemorating the recent discovery of their gene (Bergen et al. 2000; Kolata 2000; Le Saux et al. 2000; Ringpfeil et al. 2000). One speaker at the conference described PXE International as a model for other lay advocacy groups. In particular, she noted PXE International's role in engaging basic researchers and helping maintain research momentum at the same time they protected the interests and anonymity of those affected by PXE.

While the Terrys' story is unusual (and not unproblematic for the researchers with whom they work), the model they developed is becoming exemplary for other groups as they, in turn, also seek to play a role in controlling genetic research. In 2002 Pat Terry spoke at a conference of First Nations (indigenous) peoples in Vancouver, British Columbia, where he described the "PXE model," so that they, too, can adopt a proactive model of regulating scientists' access to the material products—blood, tissue, pedigrees, family studies, and gene patents—necessary for conducting their research. Here we see a dramatic example of a particular model of patient participation in the production of scientific knowledge born out of a deep desire to facilitate knowledge production on a rare genetic condition. This model highlights ordinary people not just as containers of DNA but also as producers and managers of genetic knowledge as well as potential consumers of the products that knowledge may lead to.

Like genome scientists, the Terrys are seeking a solution to a genetic condition at the molecular level. At the same time, they recognize that in order to understand what is going on at the molecular level, genetic material must be contextualized. Their personal abilities to grasp the science and to recruit and contextualize genetic material has allowed them to collaborate with researchers in pursuing their mutual desires—scientific knowledge production and a treatment for a genetic condition. And, while this is a case of a rare genetic condition, the Terrys see their work as not just a model for democratic participation in science but also as a model upon which to build the contextualizations necessary for understanding the complex pathways from structure to function. Indeed, the Terrys see themselves as mice—model organisms for understanding the complex pathways from gene to expression relevant to the more widespread common conditions in which geneticists seek to intervene.

TISSUE BANKS AND INSTITUTIONS

But, in order to understand these kinds of conditions, researchers also need access to other DNA, DNA that must also be contextualized by medical records and family histories. These efforts to materialize molecular medicine relevant to common conditions highlight both the intense desire to gain access to human biological materials and the barriers to that access. For example, researchers are now discussing their interest in mining stored tissues and medical records such as those associated with the Nurses' Health Studies.[4]

Since the specimens associated with these studies were collected "many years before the genetic revolution" (Lehman & Hohmann 2001), the forms nurses signed providing "general consent to participate in research" (Lehman & Hohmann 2001) do not say anything about genetic research. This raised questions about whether it is ethical to pursue such studies on these tissue samples. Although the consent forms signed as part of participation in these research programs did not include consent for genetic research, there now are arguments being made that these samples should be made available for molecular research without a reconsent process. The argument for this goes along these lines (and I am paraphrasing here): These are people who want to participate in research; genetic research wasn't planned when they enrolled in the research project so it isn't on the consent form; if there had been genetic research, it would have been on the consent forms, and these participants still would have been willing to sign (Lehman 2001). Nevertheless, when I asked one physician involved in this effort why, if that was the case, they didn't simply go ahead with the reconsent, she admitted, in what seems a fundamental inconsistency that "a statistically significant number might opt out" and that could damage the utility of these tissue banks.

There are also attempts to mine communities in order to develop collections of new tissue samples. Vanderbilt University and Meharry Medical

College, one of the four historically black medical colleges in the United States and one with which Vanderbilt has a joint operating agreement, are working to develop their own database of stored genetic material linked to medical records and family histories. In order to facilitate molecular research at these institutions, their administrators have decided to request a blood sample from every individual coming through either institution for any reason. The sample will be attached to their medical record, requested by their regular physician, and drawn at a time when patients are already giving blood for something else, with a blanket consent for future research.

Recognizing that informed consent for this set of practices might be rather complicated, the institution has committed to conducting community education on genetics. So here we see the "crosscutting element" of "education" in action. Reporting on this work at a conference, Ellen Clayton, a physician and lawyer involved in the project, explained that they had conducted focus groups in order "to try to understand some of the barriers [they] might experience in undergoing this process." She stated that from the focus groups, they learned that at "best a third of the people who come to our institutions might be willing to allow us to collect DNA and to allow access to medical records for purposes of research." The focus groups also indicated that, while people very much want what molecular medicine promises, "there is a deep and fundamental confusion in the population about why on earth we need DNA and medical records to do medical research." Clayton went on to explain that

> one of the things we found people saying was "If you've got my DNA, that's all there is. And so why do you need my medical records? The DNA's gonna tell you everything you need to know." Well, we know that anonymous [DNA] can't tell you everything you need to know.... [T]his is an area [where] we are really going to have to overcome public perception.

Here we see researchers running into their own prior reductivisms: Having repeatedly claimed that delineating genetic structure would lead to significant health interventions, researchers now seem surprised that people do not think more information is necessary to achieve such results.

One way the Vanderbilt-Meharry endeavor is attempting to overcome these public perceptions is through education. Vanderbilt-Meharry wants "this to be an exemplary process" in that they are attempting to "go about very seriously seeking consent and doing this in the most ethically appropriate manner." At the conference, Clayton explained that in order to "get these messages out [about] what genetic research is about and why, in fact, we need to connect DNA with medical records, and why that matters," those working at Vanderbilt-Meharry will turn "not only to the media but also to specific community events, going . . . not only to churches but also to local barbecues and other venues like that in order to talk with the population about why one wants to do this." In this way Vanderbilt-Meharry hopes to educate people so that they will be willing to participate in genetic research and also so that they will be more able to give informed consent to that participation.

The Vanderbilt-Meharry example makes clear that many people have a lot of concerns about participating in genetic research. Nevertheless, in her presentation, Clayton suggests that, although the hospitals are aware of widespread public concerns about participating in genetic research, they believe that community education will facilitate public participation. The underlying assumption here is that, if only people know what we know, they would be more willing to participate. Implicit in this assumption is the idea that concerns about participating are, by definition, the product of ignorance or confusion.

TARGETED GROUPS

In contrast to the Vanderbilt model—where education is viewed as a means to overcome concerns about genetic research—the Genetic Education for Native Americans project offers a model of education intended to enhance subjects' ability to articulate such concerns. This project is being implemented by Native American Cancer Research, an Indian owned and operated nonprofit organization, funded by the National Human Genome Research Institute and the National Institutes of Health. Here, the desire to educate people about genetics came about in reaction to requests from researchers for body tissue from Native Americans. The project aims to "provide culturally competent education about genetic research and genetic testing to Native American college and university students" (Burhanssti-panov et al. 2001). The director of the program explained to me that the goal was to provide individuals in their communities with "enough information that they can ask smart questions…so they don't get tricked."

The concern to provide people with this kind of knowledge is not simply born of a generalized distrust of the dominant society or its medical institutions. Native American Cancer Research has maintained a long-running network of breast cancer survivors' groups. When they began conducting intertribal focus groups about genetics, they learned that some members of their survivors' groups were regularly solicited for tissue samples for research and that some had been given genetic test results without any information or genetic counseling. Beyond the fact that such practices fly in the face of standard ethical practice in genetics today, this group is concerned to attend to the specific concerns people in Native American communities might have about participating in genetic research. As the director of the project explained, "[F]or some tribes some studies will be acceptable that for others will never be acceptable." When I met the director earlier this year, she elaborated on some of the reasons why some Native American communities would be unwilling to participate in genetic research no matter how well they understood its practices and purpose. These included concerns about part of the body being preserved in cell lines, about animal models, about patenting, and about migration studies. At the same time, she stressed that there are reasons why some communities might want to participate in research, particularly given serious health problems in many of these communities. The purpose of training Native American college and university students in both cultural issues and genetics is to facilitate "active, not passive informed consent" to participation in genetic research in their communities.

Another example of a community concerned about whether and how to engage genetics comes from the West Harlem Environmental Action Organization, or WE ACT—a New York City, Harlem-based activist group oriented around issues of environmental health. Since the early 1980s, there has been growing recognition in some quarters in the United States that the impact of environmental pollution disproportionately affects minority communities, leading to the development of a concept of environmental racism. WE ACT works to fight the causes of this uneven burden on poor minority communities, arguing, for example, that the increased incidence of diseases such as asthma in these communities should not be attributed to people themselves but to the environment. I was thus curious to learn that WE ACT was going to host a conference on "Genetics, the Environment, and Communities of Color" with funding from NIH/ELSI. When I attended the conference in February 2002, I learned that the conference came about because the organization's staff was increasingly encountering arguments that every medical condition, including widespread common conditions like asthma, has a genetic component that may put particular individuals at risk for developing the disease. They articulated concerns that while they needed to fight the social reasons that put members of their communities at risk, it was also important that their community not be left out of potentially beneficial health research. They held this conference, in part, as a means of educating themselves about genetics so they could evaluate the appropriateness of engaging genetic explanations for the embodied afflictions of concern in their communities. Here we find what we might call the "damned if you do, damned if you don't" model of biological citizenship. On the one hand, there is a politics of inclusion; on the other, there is the potential of displacing risk from environmental racism onto individual susceptibility and, thus, transforming environmental biopolitics into genomic biopolitics. Given NIH/ELSI's concern to gain access to certain populations' DNA, the fact that there is great interest in being able to intervene in widespread common conditions like asthma that have enormous commercial potential, and the fact that WE ACT represents a community that has a very high incidence of this condition, we have to see NIH/ELSI's interest in funding this "educational" conference as multifaceted.

There also are those who resist participating in these emerging social relations altogether. The Indigenous Peoples Council on Biocolonialism offers an interesting example of this stance. In speaking engagements, Debra Harry, the council's director, points out that the questions asked by genetic researchers are not organic to indigenous communities and do not articulate well with the interests of those communities. The council argues in its mission statement that genetic research is a new kind of colonization; that indigenous people, their blood, and their body tissue are highly desired as the objects of scientific curiosity; and that current research protections fail to recognize group rights and the rights of groups to collective control over their "collective intellectual and cultural knowledge, and genetic resources" (Indigenous Peoples Council on Biocolonialism n.d.). The organization conducts its own genetic research, which is research into the genetic research project affecting indigenous peoples, and it is engaged in a range of educational activities.

Concerns among indigenous peoples about participating in genetic research and the links made to histories of colonialism create serious issues for researchers who have continually sought access to the DNA of diverse groups since the early days of the Human Genome Project. In the early days of the Human Genome Project, a group of population geneticists and evolutionary biologists worked to establish what they called the Human Genome Diversity Project, or HGDP, through which they sought to create a databank of DNA from "isolated indigenous populations" around the world both as a means of enhancing the understanding of human evolution and in order to "preserve" human genetic diversity. In her splendid analysis of the HGDP, Jenny Reardon (2004) convincingly argues that the project failed in the United States because of researchers' apparent inability to grasp the politics of their efforts. More recent efforts to gain access to DNA from marginalized groups who may be wary of participating in medical or scientific research have been recrafted in terms of health promotion—as in the Human Genome Project's current Haplotype Map Project (U.S. National Human Genome Research Institute 2006)—or in terms of enabling people to participate in developing ancestral histories, as in the $40 million Genographic Project, a joint venture of the National Geographic Society, IBM, and the foundation supported by the Gateway Computer fortune (Pimentel 2005). Shortly after the Genographic Project was announced, the Indigenous Peoples Council on Biocolonialism called for a boycott of the project (Bio-ITWorld 2005), and the New Zealand Herald ran an article titled "Maori Alarm at Gene Project." The paper cites a researcher at Auckland University's Maori research center as stating that "this type of research is colonization as usual" ("Maori Alarm" 2005).

Like those at the Indigenous Peoples Council on Biocolonialism, Maori articulate concerns that genetic researchers conceptualize questions that may not be relevant for indigenous people. Indigenous understandings of tribal identity and origins, for example, are not linked in any obvious ways to concepts of evolution or genomics ("Maori Alarm" 2005). Similar concerns have erupted into a multimillion-dollar lawsuit brought by the Havasupai tribe of Arizona against Arizona State University (ASU) and genetic researchers there. According to the Havasupai, in 1989 they agreed to participate in a genetic study of diabetes, a condition that was of pressing concern to members of the tribe. In 2003, they learned that their DNA had been used in numerous research projects at ASU and elsewhere, including studies of schizophrenia and the peopling of the Americas, studies to which they believe they neither did provide nor would have provided consent (Hendricks 2004; Rubin 2004). One of the consequences of the Havasupai case is that numerous native groups have withdrawn consent for the use of their DNA and more than a dozen research projects involving such DNA at ASU have, thus, been shut down. Cases such as these illuminate the complicated political and ethical life of bare life in the form of DNA.

In concluding, I return to Francis Collins and his colleagues' vision of the genomic era resting firmly on the foundation of the Human Genome Project. In sketching here some of the diverse social processes aimed at materializing this genomic era, I have shown that what is going on is much more complicated than could be represented by a neat Frank Lloyd Wright–style house. For example, we might want to imagine the cross-cutting themes of resources and education as twisted together in, say, a helical-type figure. More importantly, the practices I am investigating demonstrate that far from resting on the Human Genome Project, any development of a genomic era rests on the messy border crossings and social practices involved in the emerging biopolitics of translational genomic research. It is through these practices that we see an emerging configuration of biosocial citizens whose bare life is essential for the production of knowledge and control of the health of individuals and populations and whose ethical life is being crafted as demanding participation in the knowledge production process. It is in these newly emerging biosocial assemblages upon which any genomic era will be built.

NOTES

1. Their vision of the future of genomics focuses on the need for the Human Genome Project to support biologists' access to genomic data and raw materials so biologists can develop new knowledge into not just the structure of genetic material but also, especially, its function—genomics to biology. Genomics to health is intended to facilitate health professionals' abilities to both participate in genomic research—particularly translational research that brings genetic knowledge into medical practice—and use genomic knowledge and technologies in intervening in human health. This knowledge and its associated practices, Collins and colleagues recognize, raise what they describe as "ethical, legal, and social" issues. Thus, the theme "genomics to society" focuses on the need to promote "the use of genomics to maximize benefits and minimize harms." Among the things they are concerned about

here is educating a public that can better understand "the nature and limits of genomic information" and that "grasps" its ethical, legal, and social implications.
2. Donna Haraway (2003) elaborates the idea of "an apparatus of naturalcultural production" to describe the webs of relationships across nature/culture and human/nonhuman divides through which subjects are constituted in the context of contemporary technoscience.
3. See Agamben (1998) on the concepts of bare life (*zoe*) and ethical life (*bios*). In his work *Homo Sacer*, Agamben points out that the Greeks did not have a single word for life but, rather, two: *zoe*, which referred to bare life and *bios*, which referred to ethical or political life. Agamben argues that with modernity, we see the "politicization of bare life" and that this "constitutes the decisive event of modernity" (1998: 4).
4. For history and information on the Nurses' Health Studies, some of the largest prospective studies of women's health, see Nurses' Health Study (n.d.).

REFERENCES

Agamben, Giorgio. 1995/1998. *Homo sacer: Sovereign power and bare life*, translated by Daniel Heller-Roazen. Stanford, CA: Stanford University Press.
Bergen, A., A. Plomp, E. Schuurman, S. Terry, M. Breuning, H. Dauwerse, J. Swart, M. Kook, S. van Soest, F. Baas, J. ten Brink, and P. de Jong. 2000. Mutations in ABCC6 cause Pseudoxanthoma elasticum. *Nature Genetics* 25 (June): 228–31.
Bio-ITWorld. 2005. Genographic project could repeat history. http://www-bio-itworld.com/archive/bases/042105.html (accessed November 9, 2006).
Burhansstipanov, Linda, L. Bemis, M. Bignan, C. Poodry, and F. Romero. 2001. Genetic education for Native Americans: An update and preliminary evaluation data. Paper presented at "A Decade of ELSI Research: A Celebration of the First Ten Years of the Ethical, Legal, and Social Implications (ELSI) Program," Bethesda, MD, January 17.
Collins, Francis S., Eric D. Green, Alan E. Guttmacher, and Mark S. Guyer. 2003. A vision for the future of genomics research. *Nature* 422 (April 24): 835–47.
Fortun, Michael. 2001. Mediated speculations in the genomics futures markets. *New Genetics & Society* 20, no. 2: 39–156.
Fox Keller, Evelyn 2000. *The century of the gene*. Cambridge, MA: Harvard University Press.
Fukuyama, Francis. 2002. *Our posthuman future: Consequences of the biotechnology revolution*. New York: Farrar, Straus & Giroux.
Habermas, Jürgen. 2001. On the way to liberal eugenics? The dispute over the ethical self-understanding of the species. Paper presented at the Colloquium on Law, Philosophy, and Political Theory, New York University School of Law, October 25 and November 1, New York.
Haraway, Donna. 2003. For the love of a good dog: Webs of action in the world of dog genetics. In *Race, nature, and the politics of difference*, edited by Donald S. Moore, Jake Kosek, and Anand Pandian, 254–95. Durham, NC: Duke University Press.
Hendricks 2004. Havasupai file $25M suit vs. ASU. (Flagstaff) Arizona Daily Sun, February 28. http://www.azdailysun.com/non_sec/nav_includes/story.cfm?storyID=82877&syr=2004 (accessed November 4, 2006).
Indigenous Peoples Council on Biocolonialism. n.d. http://www.ipcb.org (accessed November 9, 2006).

Kolata, G. 2000. A family's goal is met and a gene is found. *New York Times*, May 23, D2.

Lehman, Lisa. 2001. Informed consent for genetic epidemiological research. Paper presented at the Pettus-Crowe Seminar, Harvard Medical School, Division of Medical Ethics, April 27, Boston.

Lehman, Lisa, and Elizabeth Hohmann. 2001. Informed consent for genetic research in epidemiological studies. Paper presented at "A Decade of ELSI Research: A Celebration of the First Ten Years of the Ethical, Legal, and Social Implications (ELSI) Program," Bethesda, MD, January 17.

Le Saux, O., Z. Urban, C. Tschuch, K. Csiszar, B. Bacchelli, D. Quaglino, I. Pasquali-Ronchetti, F. Pope, A. Richards, S. Terry, L. Bercovitch, A. de Paepe, and C. Boyde. 2000. Mutations in a gene encoding an ABC transporter cause Pseudoxanthoma elasticum. *Nature Genetics* 25:223–27.

Maori alarm at gene project. 2005. New Zealand Herald, April 25. http://web.lexis-nexis.com/universe/document?_m=60b403e55e4983f7ccdc4d432ad0b1d8&_docnum=6&wchp=dGLbVzb-zSkVA&_md5=6af5892307fe4be43b7c19d5322a2603 (accessed August 20, 2005).

Nurses' Health Study. N.d. http://www.channing.harvard.edu/nhs (accessed November 9, 2006).

Pimentel, Benjamin. 2005. DNA study of human migration: National Geographic and IBM investigate spread of prehistoric peoples around the world. *San Francisco Chronicle*, April 13, A1.

Reardon, Jenny. 2004. *Race to the finish: Identity and governance in an age of genomics (in-formation)*. Princeton, NJ: Princeton University Press.

Ringpfeil, F., M. Lebwohl, A. Chritiano, and J. Uitto. 2000. Pseudoxanthoma elasticum: Mutations in the MRP6 gene encoding a transmembrane ATP-binding cassette (ABC) transporter. *Proceedings of the National Academy of Science* 97, no. 11: 6001–6.

Riordan, Teresa, 2002. Patents: An obsession with DNA and the human genome leads to development of a technology. *New York Times*, March 18, C2.

Rose, Hilary. 2001. Gendered genetics in Iceland. *New Genetics & Society* 20, no. 2: 119–38.

Rubin, Paul. 2004. Indian givers: The Havasupai trusted the white man to help with a diabetes epidemic. Instead, ASU tricked them into bleeding for academia. *Phoenix New Times*, May 27. http://www.phoenixnewtimes.com/issues/2004-05-27/feature.html (accessed August 20, 2006).

Sigurdsson, Skuli. 2001. Yin-yang genetics, or the HSD deCODE controversy. *New Genetics & Society* 20, no. 2: 103–17.

Specter, Michael. 1999. Decoding Iceland. *New Yorker*, January 18, 40–51.

U.S. National Human Genome Research Institute. 2006. International HapMap project. http://www.genome.gov/10001688 (accessed November 9, 2006).

12 Constructing the digital patient
Patient organizations and the development of health websites

Nelly Oudshoorn and André Somers

The Internet has become an increasingly important technology in the dissemination and use of health information (Rice & Katz 2001: 7). Since the mid-1990s, many policymakers and scholars have portrayed the Internet as a technology that changes the balance of power in the medical world in favor of the patient (Mittman & Cain 2001).[1] Patients can easily access medical information that for a long time was only available to medical professionals. They can meet and interact with doctors and other patients online, actively taking part in their diagnosis and treatment by using information from health websites (Eysenbach & Diepgen 1999; Ziebland 2004). To capture the changing relationships between patients and doctors in the "information age health care system" (Eysenbach 2000) and inspired by Giddens's notion of the reflexive consumer (Giddens 1991), sociologists have introduced new conceptualizations of patient identities, including the reflexive patient, the informed patient, the health care consumer (Eysenbach 2000), the online self-helpers (Ferguson 1997) and the net-empowered medical end-user (Ferguson 2002). This scholarship thus shows a proliferation of patient identities that challenge the earlier representations of patients as passive recipients of health care.

Although discourses on Internet and health celebrate the agency of patients, there are as yet rather few empirical studies to support this optimistic view. Recent studies have described the constraints on the emergence of the informed patient identity within patient as well as medical practitioner communities (Henwood et al. 2003). As Rice and Katz have suggested, the Internet advocates largely underestimate the realities of developing and implementing the promises of the Internet to improve and democratize health care information and communication (Rice & Katz 2001: 420). The realization of the democratic promises of the Internet is constrained by the lack of resources for the development and maintenance of digital services among many actors in the health care sector. Many health care organizations simply don't have enough funding to invest in this new technology (Mittman & Cain 2001: 60). A sustained distribution of health care information and services on the Internet requires extensive financial resources and intensive labor that may be difficult to employ for small organizations with limited funding. From this perspective, patient organizations' attempts to develop health websites are an interesting research site to understand the constraints and challenges of realizing the democratic potentials of the Internet.[2] How do these organizations, particularly those not funded by larger charities, succeed in designing websites? What are the barriers they have to overcome to gain a web presence? And, most importantly, to what extent and how do patient organizations' websites assist in the redefinition of the patient from a passive actor towards one who is an active participant in his or her care?

A second, but related, concern of our paper is to understand how patient organizations try to develop websites that are attractive and accessible for the patients they intend to reach. Or, to put it more precisely, how do patient organizations assess the interests, preferences, and digital skills of the future user of their websites? As we have described elsewhere, design practices of ICT developers are often dominated by the I-methodology: designers assume that their own preferences and skills are representative of those of the user (Rommes et al. 1999; Oudshoorn, Rommes et al. 2004; Oudshoorn, Brouns et al. 2005). The dominant rhetoric on design of ICTs has shifted from technology driven towards user-centered design, yet studies of design cultures in ICT companies in Europe show that users seem hardly to be involved in the design process, especially in the smaller ICT companies (European Commission-DG XIII-C/E 1998). In this highly competitive sector, any effort to involve users in the design is considered as a risk that may slow down the speed of development (European Commission-DG XIII-C/E 1998: 22). As nonprofits, patient organizations may reveal a different design practice because they are not under time pressure to beat the competition. Moreover, patient organizations already have an established practice of representing the patients they aim to reach. Many patient organizations have a long tradition in acting as spokespersons of patients, so we may expect that these organizations will rely on representation techniques that explicitly involve patients, rather than the I-methodology.

In this paper we analyze the design practices of three Dutch patient organizations: the Depression Foundation (Depressie Stichting), the Foundation Young People and Cancer (Stichting Jongeren en Kanker), and the Repetitive Strain Injury Patient Organization (RSI Patiëntenvereniging). We have chosen these organizations because they represent three different types of patient organizations. The Depression Foundation is a top-down organization run by health care professionals. The Foundation Young People and Cancer is a grass roots organization initiated and run by patients and their relatives. The Repetitive Strain Injury Patient Organization is a grass roots organization initiated and run by patients. The selected organizations participated in the Zon-Mw project "Patienten Organisaties, Actuele Informatie en Internet" (Patient Organizations, Timely Information and Internet), a Dutch governmental policy project aimed to support patient organizations to gain a web presence. Our study is based on an analysis of the project plans the three patient organizations developed in the context of the Zon-Mw project in which they described the aims and the content of the envisioned digital services. In addition, we have conducted interviews with representatives of the three patient organizations who have been actively involved in the development of the digital services and the project leaders of the Zon-Mw project. We also have made an analysis of the interface and the content of the digital services of the patient organizations to evaluate the extent to which they have succeeded in implementing their aims in the design of the websites. First, we describe the Dutch health care policy concerning patient organizations and Internet. The paper continues to analyze the design practices of the three patient organizations, particularly the techniques patient organizations have used to configure the user of their websites and the patient identities they constructed during the design. Finally, we will evaluate the extent to which patient organizations' websites facilitate active forms of patienthood.

DUTCH HEALTH CARE POLICY AND
THE INFORMED PATIENT

In the 1990s, Dutch policymakers articulated concerns about the quality of health care as experienced by patients (Ministerie van Volksgezondheid, Welzijn en Sport 1995). In the view of policymakers, developments in the Dutch health care system were predominantly determined by technology push incentives. They argued that the needs of end-users should become more central in making choices and setting priorities in health care (Zorg Onderzoek Nederland 1997: 7). Patients should have access to relevant information about health products and services in order to enable them to make informed choices about the care they think is most adequate for them. Dutch health care policies thus aim to contribute to the informed patient discourse. One of the organizations active in developing and implementing this policy is Zon-Mw (Health Care Research The Netherlands, Medical Sciences), a Dutch policy advisory and research organization financed by the Ministry of Health. Since the mid-1990s, this organization has developed several projects to improve the quality of information in the health care sector. According to the organization, the needs of health care consumers should play a decisive role in the choice of which information should be developed and the selection of criteria to evaluate the quality of health care products and services. Most importantly, Zon-Mw suggested that patient organizations should be considered as important groups to develop choice-supporting information from the perspective of patients (Bos & Bastiaansen 2001: 75). Equally important, the organization emphasized that the Internet could provide new opportunities to realize this aim. However, according to Dutch policymakers and Zon-Mw, there were relatively few patient organizations in The Netherlands that made optimal use of the Internet, which they mainly ascribed to the lack of human and financial resources and appropriate plans for gaining a web presence (Zon-Mw 2001a; Raad voor de Volksgezondheid & Zorg 2000).[3]

In March 2001, the organization therefore initiated the project Patienten Organisaties, Actuele Informatie en Internet (Patient Organizations, Timely Information and Internet) to support patient organizations to develop digital health services. Patient organizations were not only expected to represent and incorporate the perspective of patients, they were also expected to play an important role in providing "objective" information to counterbalance the dominance of commercial health information on the Internet (Zon-Mw 2001a: 3; interview Bastiaansen 2002). The one-year project was run by two external professionals, Lisette Bastiaansen and Renske Boersma, and consisted of several information and training sessions, including a brief Internet training session, information on the editorial and technical maintenance of websites, and advice on how to find sponsors and how to develop choice-supporting information from the perspective of the users. Patient organizations were taught several methods to use in assessing the needs and preferences of the future users of their websites, including a feedback group of end-users and testing a prototype of the website among users (Bos & Bastiaansen 2001: 37). In addition, the Zon-Mw project also offered the participating patient organizations individual support and technical assistance.

THE DEPRESSION FOUNDATION

The Depression Foundation, founded in 1995, is an organization run by a small staff bureau and volunteers, mainly psychologists, social workers, and some "experience experts" (Interview Van Geleuken & Smits 2002). The organization considers itself as the expert and major representative on the subject of depression in The Netherlands. They present the Depression Foundation as an organization of experts, not of patients (Depressie Stichting 2001a: 3). The Depression Foundation runs a phone help-desk and disseminates a flyer "Depression is a disease, not a weakness," providing information on depression. In 2001, the organization decided to join the Zon-Mw project to develop a digital Information and Advice line. The digital Information & Advice Line is the first noncommercial website on depression in the Netherlands. By creating a web presence, the Depression Foundation aims to improve the existing on- and offline information on depression. In their view, other sources often don't meet their standards of accessibility, quality, care, and continuity (Depressie Stichting 2001a).

Previous experience and i-methodology

In her seminal article on scripts, Madeleine Akrich described how designers can rely on various methods to assess the interests, competencies, and motives of future users. Following Akrich, we have analyzed the design practices of patient organizations by assessing which representation techniques dominated the design of their websites: explicit, formal representation techniques such as market surveys, consumer tests, and user feedback, or implicit, informal techniques such as reliance on expert visions, experience with other artifacts, and the I-methodology (Akrich 1995: 175).

Which representation techniques were used by the Depression Foundation to design their digital Information & Advice Line? As we described above, the Depression Foundation considers itself to be "the expert" in providing information on the topic of depression in The Netherlands. This image played an important role in the design of the structure and the content of the website. The design practice of the Depression Foundation can best be described as "design from within": to design the website, the organization relied predominantly on expertise within the organization and the I-methodology. Or, as the director and the staff member who developed the website, Ali Van Geleuken and Bianca Smits, described their design strategy: "dive into the deep and see what happens." Instead of trying to assess the needs of the future users by explicit representation techniques, the staff members relied heavily on the I-methodology:

> In everything we offer on the website, we have tried to think from the perspective of the target group. We have done this together, just the two of us sitting in front of the computer and giving comments to each other.... In this way we developed our own style. (Interview Van Geleuken & Smits 2002)

The staff members of the Depression Foundation considered the ICT project as "their project": they wanted to learn from the project before they shared their experiences with other people in the organization or had to deal with feedback by users to be sure that "it became the project we wanted it to be" (Interview Geleuken & Smit 2002). For example, the decision that a flat navigation structure[4] of the interface of the website would be better for people suffering from depression because of their concentration problems, and that this should be implemented in the design of the website by offering all information on the front page with few clicks to other pages (Depressie Stichting 2001b: 1; interview Van Geleuken & Smits 2002), had not been tested among depression patients. As we will learn from the design practices of the Foundation Young People and Cancer, there are other ways in which the structure of the interface can be organised to cater to the needs of users with concentration problems.

The design from within strategy was also used to develop the content of the website. The staff members used their own professional expertise in the area of psychology and psychiatry and the expertise of members of the board, all health care professionals, as the main input to decide on the content of the website. In addition to relying on their own knowledge and expert knowledge within the organization, the staff members relied on another implicit representation technique: experience with other artifacts.

To develop the content of the website, Van Geleuken and Smits used data they had collected on the users of the phone help desk and the information leaflet of the Depression Foundation: "Depression Is a Disease, Not a Weakness" (Depressie Stichting 2001a: 9). They largely copied the content and design characteristics of this leaflet (Interview Van Geleuken & Smits 2002). Explicit methods that were suggested by the project leaders of the Zon-Mw project as relevant design strategies for the development of the website, such as formal user tests and feedback groups consisting of patients, were not used. The Depression Foundation decided to postpone the testing to the use phase: they planned to improve the website in reaction to experiences of users.

Summarizing, we can conclude that the design practice of the Depression Foundation is very similar to the design practices of small ICT firms we described above: the organization predominantly relied on in-house experience and did not consult any future users. To realize the final phase of the development of the website, the Depression Foundation hired an experienced web designer to build the website. The website of the organization can thus be considered as a coproduction of the director, the staff member, and an IT expert from outside the organization.

Configuring the user as patient

The design from within strategy resulted in a construction of the identity of the future users of the website in which the image of the user conflated with representations of the disorder. Based on their knowledge of depression, the director and the staff member constructed the user of their website as a patient who suffers from a severe depression: users are considered to be "isolated, distrustful, undecided, introvert, fearful, and uncertain" (Depressie Stichting 2001a: 2). The form and content of the website of the Depression Foundation show that the image of the user as someone who suffers from a severe depression played an important role in guiding the design, particularly choices concerning the provision of interactive parts.[5] The website of the organization includes general information about the Depression Foundation; information about several types of depressions and therapies that can be downloaded from the web page; a section called "frequently asked questions"; a section called "personal advice" consisting of a form where users can ask for information or help; a test for self-diagnosis; and a forum for relatives of people who suffer from depression. Interactive facilities for patients, such as a forum, mail groups, or chat rooms, are not included. Although the Depression Foundation has considered including a chat room moderated by a psychiatrist, the organization decided to restrict the interactive parts of the websites to relatives of patients. Contacts between people who suffer from severe depression were considered too risky: exchange of experiences and advice by patients was expected to have a negative impact because it would lower their spirits (Interview Van Geleuken & Smits 2002). The image of the user as a patient who suffers from a severe depression thus resulted in the exclusion of patients' experience-based knowledge.

In other parts of the website, this representation of the user was not used as a guideline for the design. Although the Depression Foundation aimed to develop a calm and sober website with a flat navigation structure because people who suffer from depression have problems with concentration, these requirements were not implemented in the design. The navigation structure used for information on different types of depression is deeper than necessary and references in the text are difficult to find. Hyperlinks (i.e. words and pictures on a page that can make it easier to find other relevant information on the website), are little used. Moreover, the form on the website where people who visit the website can ask for personal advice, offers a very limited space (24×4 characters) for users to present their question. The format of the form makes it rather difficult to articulate a carefully formulated request. Finally, the texts consist of rather long and complex sentences. Consequently, the use of the website requires quite some concentration and therefore does not cater to the needs of the patient with depression as articulated by the Depression Foundation. In this respect, the organization has failed to attune the design of the website to the conditions of patients suffering from severe depression.

THE FOUNDATION YOUNG PEOPLE AND CANCER

The Foundation Young People and Cancer (Stichting voor Jongeren en Kanker) is a small organization founded by relatives of young people with cancer and run by volunteers, including (ex) cancer patients and their relatives. They aim to give psychosocial support to young people with cancer (15–35 years) following their medical treatment, and emphasize the importance of timely care for nonsomatic aspects of cancer. The organization's major activities consist of the organization of weekends for patients to socialize and relax, meetings to facilitate contacts for companions in distress, and informative meetings with experts (Stichting Jongeren en Kanker 2002a: 4, 6, 18).

In 2001, the Foundation Young People and Cancer initiated the Internet Harbor (Internet Haven). The Internet Harbor project consisted of the development of a website and a CD-ROM. The name is carefully chosen to articulate the aim of this digital project: "to offer a digital beacon of safety and security" to young people with cancer (Zon-Mw 2001b). The organization initiated the digital project because of "the lack of timely help with respect to vital questions and practical problems such as schools and insurance" (Stichting Jongeren en Kanker 2002a: 2).

The creation of digital services is an important development for the Foundation Young People and Cancer. Due to Internet presence the organization is more widely known and its membership has increased (Interview Van der Wal 2002). Although the Foundation for Young people and Cancer is a small patient organization, the Internet Harbor project can be considered as an important contribution to the provision of online patient-oriented, and noncommercial information and care for young cancer patients. All the other Dutch websites on youth cancer are commercial sites, except for the website of the Vereniging voor Ouders van Kinderen met Kanker (Society for Parents of Children with Cancer) (Interview Van der Wal 2002).

Expert visions and user feedback

Like the Depression Foundation, the Foundation Young People and Cancer used a variety of representation techniques. All through the project, the Advisory Council of the organization played an important role in guiding the design of the Internet Harbor project. The professional expertise of its members, including psychologists, psychiatrists, and oncologists, and a textbook written by one of the psychologists on psychosocial patient care in oncology, were used as major resources to develop the first ideas on the content of the website (Interview Elzinga 2002). The organization thus relied on expert ideas, including in-house expertise as well as the expertise of other organizations that specialized in pediatric oncology and patient care.

Another implicit representation technique used to develop their digital project consisted of the experience and knowledge the project leader Van der Wal had gained from intensive interactions with young cancer patients, both on- and offline. By following the discussions among patients on mailing lists of another website which he had initiated for cancer patients (diagnosekanker.nl), the project leader became familiar with what was going on among cancer patients. Van der Wal used these mailing lists to ask the participants what they considered to be relevant information. In a later phase, the mailing lists were also used to test the organization's pilot website (Interview Van der Wal 2002). As a grass roots organization, the Foundation Young People and Cancer could also rely on the contacts they had established with young cancer patients. Discussions with patients and their relatives during the social activities organized by the organization were used as major resources to decide on the topics that should be included on the website (Interview Elzinga 2002). Patient knowledge and preferences have played an important role in the development of the organization's digital services.

In addition to these implicit representation techniques, the Foundation Young People and Cancer also applied the explicit methods of user feedback and consumer testing. At the beginning of the digital project, the organization initiated the Youth Team, a group of 10–12 (ex)cancer patients who were invited to participate in the project by personal contacts and a call on the website diagnosiscancer.nl (Stichting Jongeren en Kanker 2002a: 22; Interview Elzinga 2002). The organization thus implemented the advice of the Zon-Mw project leaders to install a feedback group that represented the target group. Members of the Youth Team were asked to evaluate the content of the website and the CD-ROM and to indicate and articulate the shortcomings of the pilot website. The Foundation Young People and Cancer also conducted several tests among potential users, including members of the Youth team to collect feedback on the initial design of the website and the CD-ROM.

The development of the digital services of the Foundation for Young People and Cancer exemplifies a design practice in which both experts and patients played an important role. Compared to the Depression Foundation, the Foundation Young People and Cancer has shown a more democratic design culture in which patients were invited to act as advisors and test-users. The way in which the organization launched their digital services is another illustration of this design culture. In March 2002, the Foundation Young People and Cancer organized a kick-off meeting with members of the board, the advisory council, the Youth Team, and the volunteers to involve them in the project. Or, as the invitation for the meeting suggested: "we want to use your talents as best as we can in a way that fits your interests" (Stichting Jongeren en Kanker 2002b). A similar meeting was organized at the end of the project where all groups were invited on a boat trip to symbolize the successful completion of the Internet Harbor project.

Designing for patients with psycho-social problems and physical constraints

The involvement of experts and patients in the development of the digital services resulted in the construction of the identity of the future user of the digital services of the Foundation Young People and Cancer as a young cancer patient who is at risk of having specific psychosocial problems. The digital services should cater for the needs of young cancer patients who can become isolated after their medical treatment if they don't succeed in finding the way to psychosocial care (Interview Van der Wal 2002). Based on this image of the future user, the organization introduced the metaphor of the Internet harbor. The harbor metaphor was used as a guideline for the graphic design of the website. Instead of a "wild" design, the Foundation for Young People and Cancer preferred a calm, pleasant interface to offer a feeling of safety (Interview Tom van de Wal 2002). Other important aspects in configuring the user were the mental and physical constraints experienced by cancer patients. According to the organization, (young) people with cancer suffer from a lack of concentration and energy resulting from the medical treatment, particularly chemotherapy. A calm design should therefore also include an easy-to-use navigational structure (Interview Van der Wal 2002).

The Foundation Young People and Cancer thus reflects a similar design strategy to that of the Depression Foundation: both organizations aimed to develop a website that should not be too demanding for people with concentration problems. However, the two organizations chose completely opposite ways to translate this user requirement into the design of their respective websites. Whereas the Depression Foundation opted for a so-called flat structure, which resulted in more text on one page, the Foundation Young People and Cancer chose a deep structure with relatively short texts on one page (Interview Van der Wal 2002). These different technological choices illustrate that there is no uniform, standardized approach to cater to the needs of future users with concentration problems.

The design practices of the Foundation for Young People and Cancer also show that it is not always an easy job to translate user requirements into the design of digital services. Although the organization put quite some effort in trying to assess the needs and skills of the future user of their digital services, they have been less successful in integrating these requirements in the design of the website. Due to the graphic design and inconsistencies in the navigation structure, the website does not have the calm and safe image the organization preferred. The graphic design is such that the texts are put on pictures as background, which make the letters less sharp and makes it impossible to enlarge the text and to provide hyperlinks to other pages. Inconsistencies in the design of the pages and the references to other pages offered in the texts further complicate the use of the website.

Although the Foundation Young People and Cancer thus failed in translating the image of the user as a patient at risk of isolation and suffering from concentration problems into the structure of the website, the organization was more effective in incorporating this image in the type of services they have developed. The organization realized several facilities to diminish the risk that young people with cancer become isolated. "Mutual support among patients" was used as a key term in the design of the content and the services. The website of the organization therefore includes mailing groups and a log book to facilitate contacts between patients. Exchange of experiences and information among young people with cancer is considered as crucial for the empowerment of patients. Or to quote the project leader Van der Wal: "problems can often be solved in groups of 'companions in distress', simply because they recognize each others problems" (Interview Van der Wal 2002). The actual use of the website shows that the log book function is used very frequently, providing new stories of patients almost every day.[6] Another important guiding principle that the organization realized in the design of their digital services is that patients can recover best if they can play an active role themselves (Stichting Jongeren en Kanker 2002a: 4, 6). The organization considers the active involvement of patients in the treatment process as beneficial for the recovery and effective in diminishing problems in coping with the disease. To facilitate this form of self-care, the CD-ROM included a module on psychosocial care and social services that supports patients in choosing the type of care they think they need. Moreover, the website offers a digital diary, in which patients can record their own experiences with their disease, and a digital buddy: a virtual (ex)patient who is available for personal advice and support. The Foundation for Young People and Cancer thus provides a wider variety of digital services to facilitate mutual support among patients and self-care than the Depression Foundation.

THE RSI PATIENT ORGANIZATION

The RSI patient organization, founded in 1995, is a grass roots organization initiated and run by volunteers diagnosed with repetitive strain injury. The organization profiles itself as "the independent, objective, and non-commercial information source about RSI" (RSI Patiëntenvereniging 2002: 1, 2). The RSI patient organization has a phone help-desk and publishes a quarterly journal. It is run by approximately 60 volunteers, mainly women who, before their illness, used to work in highly qualified computer jobs. Most of these volunteers are constrained in what they can actually do for the organization because they suffer from RSI. In 2001, the organization decided to join the Zon-MW project and to develop a new website.[7]

Experience-based knowledge and informal methods

For the development of the new website, the RSI patient organization relied primarily on experience-based knowledge. As a grass roots organization, they had easy access to expertise on RSI provided by the volunteers, all people with RSI or ex-RSI patients. Volunteers were not only useful resources because of their experience-based knowledge with RSI, they also provided in-house expertise with computers and Internet technology. To enroll the volunteers' expertise, the RSI patient organization initiated an advisory group, consisting of volunteers with expertise on the design of interfaces and other aspects of Internet technology. In addition, the organization formed an advisory committee that, according to the project plan, should have the responsibility to control and monitor the quality of the information on the website (RSI Patiëntenvereniging 2002: 5). In addition to using the in-house experience of the volunteers and the advisory committee, the project leader also relied on the I-methodology. To decide on what topics are relevant to include in the website, the project leader used his own expertise as an ex-RSI patient: "You try to imagine what type of questions will be asked and what problems actually exist" (Interview Jan Wassenaar 2002). In addition, he relied on what he knew about the organization's experience with its telephone service for RSI patients. However, this source of information was not used in a systematic way.

The design practice was thus dominated by a mixture of informal methods to assess the needs and preferences of users. Explicit representation techniques such as formal user tests or surveys among future users were not applied. The organization has planned to involve users to evaluate and improve the website once it is in use and in the second phase of the digital project when the development of the interactive parts of the website takes place. Reflecting on the first phase of the design practice of the RSI patient organization, we can conclude that this organization reveals a design culture similar to the Depression Foundation. Both organizations relied on implicit representation techniques and did not use any formal methods to assess the needs of users. However, there is a major difference between the two organizations. The reliance on informal methods by the Depression Foundation resulted in a prioritization of expert knowledge because the director and the staff member in charge of the digital project were professionals and not patients. For the RSI patient organization the reliance on the I-methodology resulted in a privileging of experience-based knowledge.

Like the Depression Foundation, the RSI patient organization decided to hire people to assist them to build the website, in this case a professional web designer and a journalist. This choice seems rather peculiar because the organization could have used its in-house experience with Internet technology. However, they preferred to hire an experienced web designer because of their negative experience with the first website. Moreover, by choosing to hire people from outside the organization, they could avoid time-consuming discussions among the volunteers who all had their own preferences and skills as IT workers. The website was thus realized by a collective effort of the project leader, some volunteers, and two professional employees. The expertise of the volunteers was used as a resource to compile a very detailed list of technical specifications, including requirements to facilitate an easy-to-use navigation structure and other standards of accessibility that were used as guideline for the design of the website.

Imaging users as active patients and users of the internet

The reliance on the in-house experience of the volunteers and the project leader resulted in a mixture of patient identities. According to the project leader, people with RSI are "perfectionist people who make high demands and are sensitive to stress" (Interview Wassenaar 2002). This image of the patient merges with another identity: RSI patients are portrayed as very active Internet users (RSI Patiëntenvereniging 2002). At first sight, the latter image of the user may be considered as a problematic identity because frequent use of the computer can be the very cause of the disease. However, the RSI patient organization expected that RSI patients would use the Internet to find relevant information about their disease because they are very familiar with this technology. Most importantly, they have tried to implement several measures to enable RSI patients to use their website efficiently. In the project plan, the organization emphasized that the website should have a sober and user friendly design with "short and simple navigation routes," and avoid any unnecessary gadgets (RSI Patiëntenvereniging 2002: 9, 18). "A few clicks should be enough to find the relevant information" (Interview Wassenaar 2002). The eventual form of the website illustrates that the organization has been rather successful in realizing these aims. Most specifications included in the list of requirements we described earlier have been implemented in the design. The website contains a short and clear navigation structure, avoiding any unnecessary deep structures, and it provides easy-to-read texts consisting of short paragraphs and rather simple sentences.

Like the Foundation Young People and Cancer, the RSI patient organization chose to exploit the new possibilities of Internet, particularly its interactive facilities. The image of the user as an active, informed patient has been used as guideline for the design. The website includes a mailing list where users can post messages to exchange information and experiences with specific therapies and other relevant topics. To cater to the needs of RSI patients, the organization has also developed and introduced specific norms of behavior for the users of their mailing list, a so-called netiquette. Compared to other mailing lists, that usually encourage the use of correct and complete sentences, correct punctuation, and the avoidance of abbreviations, the RSI accepts the frequent use of abbreviations and does not ask the user to use capital letters.[8] In addition, users of the mailing list are not expected to correct any typing errors. These divergent norms are introduced to diminish the barriers for RSI patients to send messages to the mailing list. The development of this netiquette shows how the RSI patient organization has found a creative way to adapt their website to the needs of people with RSI. However, the other interactive facilities the organization had planned to develop, such as a discussion forum and the exchange and collection of the website users' experience-based knowledge, have not been realized yet because of financial and manpower constraints. The maintenance of the website, including the responsibility to keep the information up-to-date, is considered a priority.

CONCLUSIONS

Reflecting on our case studies, we can conclude that the democratic potential of the Internet is not inherent capacity in the new technology but requires hard work. As we have described in the introduction, the development and maintenance of websites to spread sustained information via the Internet requires resources that many people and organizations such as small patient collectives simply don't have. The Internet can thus be considered as a technology that adds to the already existing barriers and challenges posed to patient organizations more generally when they try to realize democratic potentials (Epstein 1996). Our research illustrates that patient organizations have to overcome specific barriers to develop digital services. Although the three organizations we studied received considerable support from the Zon-Mw organization, they nevertheless faced certain constraints that had negative consequences for the plans they wanted to realize. Lack of financial resources and manpower were the main reasons why the RSI patient organization had to postpone the development of interactive parts of their website. Even the Depression Foundation, the organization that had been successful in getting enough funding to start a website, had to decide to stop the personal advice services on their website because of the costs and the work involved in providing this service. Other barriers the patient organizations had to overcome included access to digital expertise to build the websites. Our analysis of the three patient organizations thus shows that the development of a website is a very demanding task, even for patient organizations that have in-house expertise with computers and the Internet.

In contrast to what Zon-Mw and the authors of the present paper expected, patient organizations don't consider the involvement of patients as crucial for the design of health websites: two of the three organizations primarily relied on informal representation techniques, particularly the I-methodology. As for other organizations, the I-methodology should be considered to be an inadequate design methodology because it excludes the perspectives and needs of people with other demographic characteristics than those of the designer. Studies of projects in which patients were explicitly involved in setting up a website (Parr 2001) or invited to present their experiences, show patient-centered methods as being very adequate in developing websites that meet patients' information needs (Rosmovits & Ziebland 2004). In the case of patient organizations, the lack of user involvement cannot be explained in terms of economic incentives such as time pressure to beat the competition, as has been described for commercial organizations (European Commission-DG XIII-C/E 1998). Instead we suggest that the extent to which patient organizations involve users in the design of their websites should be ascribed to previously established routines and practices of representing patients within the organizations. The only organization that invited patients to participate in the design of their digital services, the Foundation Young People and Cancer, had strong relations with patients because of the social events they frequently organize for young people with cancer. In contrast, the other two organizations did not have any established contacts with patients. Consequently, they did not make any attempts to involve users in the design, and postponed user feedback. Our research thus confirms previous research findings that users, in this case patients, are largely absent from the design process of information and communication technologies (Mort et al. 2003; Rommes et al. 1999; Oudshoorn, Rommes et al. 2004; Oudshoorn, Brouns et al. 2005).

In our paper we also tried to explore the extent to which patient organizations' websites assist in redefining the patient from passive recipient to active participant in his or her care. If we take the two aspects identified in the literature on the active patient model, as criteria, maximization of self-care and increased independence from health professionals (Kendall 2001), the following picture emerges. All three organizations, although there are major differences between them, have developed websites that support self-care and might encourage independence from health professionals. The Depression Foundation has included a self-diagnosis test on their website that enables patients to make a diagnosis of their psychological problems and to learn about relevant therapies. Although the Depression Foundation's website thus facilitates active forms of patienthood, it also sets limits to the active patient model: mutual support among patients themselves is considered as disempowering. Therefore the organization has not included interactive facilities for patients on their website. Consequently, the website does not support the exchange of experience-based knowledge; for example, how patients and their relatives can learn to cope with depression and this diminishes the possibilities for self-care. As recent studies have indicated, patients highly value experiential information from other patients (Rosmovits & Ziebland 2004).

The digital services of the Foundation Young People and Cancer offer two facilities to support self-care: choice-supporting information about psychosocial care and a digital diary. The organization also facilitates mutual support among patients by providing mail groups and a discussion forum where patients can exchange experiences and information. Moreover, they provide alternative health services by introducing the digital buddy who can give personal advice and support. These services can contribute to making patients less dependent on health care professionals. In contrast to the Depression Foundation, the Foundation Young People and Cancer thus exploits the interactive facilities of the new technology to encourage mutual support and self-care. Although the organization provides new services that facilitate active forms of patienthood, the organization remains, however, within the scope of activities characteristic for traditional patient organizations: they adhere to a strict distribution of roles between patient organizations and health professionals.[9] The Foundation Young People and Cancer only deals with psychosocial aspects of cancer; the medical expertise remains defined as the domain of specialists (doctors and researchers). The organization does not claim to play a role in changing or criticizing the health care system, neither does it aim to contribute to the production of expert knowledge on cancer.

Finally, the website of the RSI patient organization provides information on different aids for prevention of RSI and recovery, thus supporting self-care. Like the Foundation Young People and Cancer, the RSI patient organization considers the interactive facilities of websites as important tools for patients' empowerment. Their website includes a mailing list for patients and they have planned to develop other interactive parts to collect experience-based knowledge to evaluate the quality of care available for RSI patients and gain new knowledge of the disease. As we have described above, these plans have been postponed because of lack of financial resources and manpower. Nevertheless, the organization's intentions indicate that the RSI patient organization uses the Internet as a tool to extend its activities beyond the traditional role of patient organizations; they aim to contribute to the construction of knowledge on the disease, a role that is usually delegated to scientists. Summarizing, we can conclude that patient organizations' digital services facilitate active forms of patienthood. The extent to which these websites will eventually function as tools to encourage a balanced encounter between patients and health professionals remains, however, in the hands of the patients and their doctors.

NOTES

Acknowledgments. We would like to thank Onno Elzinga, Ali Van Geleuken, Bianca Smits, Tom Van der Wal, and Jan Wassenaar for their detailed accounts of their experiences in developing the digital services of their organizations, and Lisette Bastiaansen and Renske Boersma for sharing their experiences with the Zon-MW project.

   This article has been published in *Information, Communication & Society* 2006, 9, 5: 657–75 (http://www.tandf.co.uk/journals), and is reprinted with kind permission of the Taylor & Francis Group.

1. Earlier versions of this paper have been presented at the EASST conference in York 2002, the 4S conference in Milwaukee 2002, and the workshop on Patient Organizations in Göteborg, June 2003.
2. To be sure, we don't suggest that all patient organizations face similar financial barriers. Patient organizations funded by larger charities, particularly in the areas of cancer and heart disease, are often well funded and have developed websites with high hit rates.
3. Two of the three patient organizations we studied, the Foundation Young People and Cancer and the Repetitive Strain Injury Patient Organization, receive funding from the Patient Fund, the Dutch governmental funding agency for patient organizations. The Depression Foundation is not funded by the Patient Fund because the organization is not considered to be a patient organization since it is not initiated and run by patients (Interview Geleuken and Smits 2002).
4. The navigation structure of a website is the way in which the individual pages are ordered and the linkages between them. This structure provides the route by means of which the user can assess the information provided on the different pages.
5. Our analysis of the website is based on the version that was available on January 6, 2003.
6. Although the log book function is frequently used, the number of people using this function is rather low.
7. In contrast to the other two organizations, the RSI patient organization had already launched a website which they considered to be "not professional" (Interview Wassenaar, 2002). It was only due to the support of the Zon-Mw project that the RSI organization could take the step of developing a website that met their standards for adequate digital support of RSI patients.
8. The use of the shift key required for capital letters is considered as problematic for RSI patients.
9. As Barbot (2006) has described, most patient organizations that were initiated in the 1950s and 1960s and 1970s, restricted their activities to improving the everyday situation of patients and focused their attention on the psycho-

social aspects of diseases. According to Barbot, this distribution of roles was first criticized in the early 1980s when patient collectives began to include an active involvement with medical knowledge and research in their agenda.

REFERENCES

Akrich, Madeleine 1995. User representations: Practices, methods and sociology. In *Managing technology in society: The approach of constructive technology assessment*, edited by A. Rip, T. J. Misa, and J. Schot, 167–84. London: Pinter.

Barbot, Janine. 2006. How to build an active patient? The work of AIDS associations in France. *Social Science and Medicine*, 62, no.3: 538–51.

Bastiaansen, Lisette. 2002. (Interview). Coordinator of the project 'Patiënten Organisaties, Actuele Informatie en Internet' (Patient Organizations, Timely Information and Internet) initiated by Zorg Onderzoek Nederland—Medische Wetenschappen (Health Care Research The Netherlands — Medical Sciences). February 19.

Boersma, Renske. 2002. (Interview). Coordinator of the project 'Patiënten Organisaties, Actuele Informatie en Internet' (Patient Organizations, Timely Information and Internet) initiated by Zorg Onderzoek Nederland—Medische Wetenschappen (Health Care Research The Netherlands — Medical Sciences). February 19.

Bos, R., and L. Bastiaansen. 2001. *Patientenorganisaties, actuele informatie en internet. Programma-overzicht (plenaire bijeenkomsten en individuele begeleiding) en dagprogramma's (plenaire bijeenkomsten)*. Den Haag: Zon-Mw.

Depressie Stichting. 2001a. Projectplan voor de realisatie van het internetproject van ZON. Projectplan Depressie Stichting.

———. 2001b. Bijlage opzet en structuur website. Projectplan Depressie Stichting.

Elzinga, Onno. 2002. (Interview). Chairman of the board of the Foundation Young People and Cancer (Stichting Jongeren en Kanker). February 21.

Epstein, Steven. 1996. *Impure science: AIDS, activism, and the politics of knowledge*. Berkeley: University of California Press.

European Commission- DG XIII-C/E. 1998. Telematics applications programme "Design for All" for an inclusive information society. In *Design for All and ICT Business practice*. EC reference no. 98.70.022.

Eysenbach, Gunther. 2000. Consumer health informatics. *British Medical Journal* 320:1713–16.

Eysenbach, Gunther, and Thomas L. Diepgen. 1999. Patients looking for information on the Internet and seeking teleadvice. *Journal of American Medical Association* 135:151–56.

Ferguson, Tom. 1997. Health online and the empowered medical consumer. *Journal of Quality Improvement* 23, no. 5: 251–57.

———. 2002. From patients to end users. Quality of online patient networks needs more attention than quality of online health information. *British Medical Journal* 334:556–57.

Giddens, Anthony. 1991. *Modernity and self-identity*. Oxford: Polity.

Henwood, Flis, Sally Wyatt, Angie Hart, and Julie Smith. 2003. Ignorance is bliss sometimes: Constraints on the emergence of the "informed patient" in the changing landscapes of health information. *Sociology of Health and Illness* 25, no. 6 (September): 589.

Kendall, Liz. 2001. *The future patient*. London: Institute for Public Policy Research.

Ministerie van Volksgezondheid, Welzijn en Sport. 1995. Beleidsbrief Patienten/consumentenbeleid in de Zorgsector. Den Haag: Ministerie van VWS.

Mittman, Robert, and Mary Cain. 2001. The future of the Internet in health care. In *The Internet and health communication: Experiences and expectations,* edited by R. E. Rice and J. E. Katz, 47–75. Thousand Oaks, CA: Sage.

Mort, Maggie, Carl R. May, and Tracy Williams. 2003. Remote doctors and absent patients: Acting at a distance in telemedicine? *Science, Technology & Human Values* 28, no. 2: 274–96.

Oudshoorn, Nelly, Margo Brouns, and Ellen van Oost. 2005. Diversity and distributed agency in the design and use of medical video-communication technologies. In *Inside the politics of technology: Agency and normativity in the co-production of technology and society,* edited by H. Harbers. Amsterdam: Amsterdam University Press.

Oudshoorn, Nelly, Els Rommes, and Marcelle Stienstra. 2004. Configuring the user as everybody: Gender and cultures of design in information and communication technologies. *Science, Technology & Human Values* 29, no. 1: 30–64.

Parr, S. P. 2001. Inclusive Internet technologies for people with communication impairment. Stroke News: Stroke Association, September.

Raad voor de Volksgezondheid & Zorg. 2000. *Patient en Internet, advies uitgebracht door de Raad voor de Volksgezondheid en Zorg aan de minister van Volksgezondheid, Welzijn en Sport.* Zoetermeer: Raad voor de Volksgezondheid en Zorg.

Rice, Ronald E., and James E. Katz. 2001. *The Internet and health communication: Experiences and expectations.* Thousand Oaks, CA: Sage.

Rommes, Els, Ellen van Oost, and Nelly Oudshoorn. 1999. Gender and the design of a digital city. Information, *Communication and Society* 2, no. 4: 476–95.

Rosmovits, Linda, and Sue Ziebland. 2004. What do patients with prostate cancer or breast cancer want from an Internet site? A qualitative study of information needs. *Patient Education and Counseling* 53:57–64.

RSI Patiëntenvereniging. 2002. RSI-patiënten: van shoppen naar kiezen—projectplan voor keuzeondersteunende informatie over RSI en Internet, projectplan voor de realisatie van het internetproject van ZON. http://www.rsi-vereniging.nl (accessed October 30, 2006).

Smits, Bianca. 2002. (Interview). Staffmember at the Depression Foundation (Depressie Stichting). June 3.

Stichting Jongeren en Kanker. 2002a. Project internethaven. Plan en realisatie, projectplan voor de realisatie van het internetproject van ZON.

———. 2002b. Uitnodiging kick off Internet haven.

van Geleuken, Ali. 2002. (Interview). Staffmember at the Depression Foundation (Depressie Stichting). June 3.

van der Wal, Tom. 2002. (Interview). Project coordinator at the Foundation Young People and Cancer (Stichting Jongeren en Kanker). February 19.

Wassenaar, Jan. 2002. (Interview). Volunteer at the Repetitive Strain Injury Patient Organization (RSI patienten vereniging). June 29.

Ziebland, Sue 2004. The importance of being expert: The quest for cancer information on the Internet. *Social Science and Medicine* 59:1783–93.

Zon-Mw. 2001a. Nieuwsbrief Consumenteninformatie. Special Consumenteninformatie op Internet. *Jaargang* 5, no. 4. Den Haag: Zon-Mw.

———. 2001b. *Overzicht van de project plannen.* June. Den Haag: Zon-Mw.

Zorg Onderzoek Nederland. 1997. *Informatie op Koers.* Den Haag: Zon-Mw.

Epilogue
Indeterminate lives, demands, relations: Emergent bioscapes

Joseph Dumit and Regula Valérie Burri

Biomedicine as Culture is a collection of contemporary anthropology and related work that addresses the postgenomic, postmedical, postindividual world as we will discuss it below. The convergence of new life tech, info tech, industrialized life sciences, and corporate clinical trials has created what Michael Fischer (2003) calls an ethical plateau—stratified situations where uncertainties accumulate while decisions must be made. The topics of this book—genetic testing, uncertain high-tech knowledges, medicalization in the wake of patient activism, and interactive bodily construction and maintenance—are such plateaus. Let us call this uneven terrain our bioscape. The essays in this volume each track emergent, tentative, declarative, improper solutions. This list of contradictory adjectives is an empirical finding: Decisions regarding the use of an Alzheimer's screening test based on incomplete information, decisions regarding the use of blood obtained from experiments 40 years ago used today for genetic tests, and decisions to keep bone marrow donors and recipients from knowing each other: These decisions declare that the sociality of people can be changed the next day on grounds of evidence, morals, politics, law, lawsuits, or experiments. These decisions, in other words, are themselves part of experimental systems in Rheinberger's (1997) sense, continually defining and revising their objects, their rationality, their purpose, and their past.

In this epilogue, we want to sketch some features of this bioscape that are shared across the ethical plateaus being studied. The first feature is the postgenomic crisis of indetermination. Many of the articles reference Evelyn Fox Keller's (2000) analysis of the twentieth century as the century of the gene for its cogent summary of a field of promises that continues to remain unfulfilled. What had been from conception a fetish and a fantasy of control—the gene as an informatic transmitter of heredity—produced instead a layered series of deferrals and guesses. We now have "tests" "for" "genes" "for" "Alzheimer's." The necessity to put each of these words in quotation marks underscores the problem of uncertainty relating to determining the objects—tests, genes, disease-syndromes—and the relations between them. In so many different ways, we have too much information to the point of excess, and at the same time not enough. Overdetermination and underdetermination combine to produce indetermination. And it is often the indeterminate result which is then handed over to the patient for their choice and consent, in a mockery of both information and responsibility.

Growing up alongside the molecular revolution was the computer industry and the very possibility of crunching the numbers and manipulating the mass scale of the microbiology necessary to sequence the genome, create the MRI, and manage 10,000+ person clinical trials. One consistent demand of the information technologies is the standardization and comparability of life, bodies, and subjects. Lock, for instance, finds that the uncertainties in the experimental system of Alzheimer's disease (AD) nonetheless increasingly put people in only one of three boxes of disease futures via a relatively simple set of criteria. Burri looks at how technological constraints and standardization infuse the entire MRI suite at the level of anatomy: Not only do MRIs normalize patients to referent anatomical atlases (Beaulieu 2001), but their architecture and clinical organization also imply a sociotechnical anatomy which generates patients according to their size, metal content, and psychic ability to follow directions and withstand claustrophobic conditions. This sociotechnical anatomy is the corollary of any info-biotechnology that coordinates biology, subjectivity, workflow, and throughput.

Schubert explores a related info-bio process, the operating room. He approaches it through an ethnographic perspective on nurses and anesthetists. These two participants in the complex of monitoring devices, patients, anesthesia, and operating room architecture must negotiate, coordinate, and adjust to the myriad "glitches" that afflict treatment. As Elizabeth Roberts (1998) has shown regarding electronic fetal monitors, info-bio monitoring devices introduced into health situations can take over attention, structuring patient care to their own rhythm, and even come to redefine standards of care. Schubert discusses how the torrent of information, especially alarms on various devices, must be learned in order to be managed. He attends to how nurses often become key mentors in teaching new anesthetists what part of the excessive inputs they must coordinate to, and what parts might be turned off.

Oudshoorn and Somers look at a third type of info-bio interface, the Internet seen as a coordinating site for patients, information, experts, and sociality. Looked at from the perspective of website designers, the authors compare vastly different approaches of constructing visitors as users, and users as patients. With an eye toward participatory design ideas, they suggest ways in which some designs actively contribute to sociality and lateral sharing, and others reinforce hierarchical notions of experts and information flow. Importantly, Oudshoorn and Somers show how the composition of the design teams themselves mirrors the site design philosophies adopted. We think this insight is crucial for the entire bioscape, raising the following question: What sorts of teams design the MRI suites, the OR and monitors, clinical trials, genetic research protocols, counseling exams, and organ donation practices? How might these be designed differently according to different notions of participation?

Taussig addresses these questions for informed consent. Examining the transformation of consent from a one-way acknowledgment of possible harm to a two-way contract, she shows how patient groups, indigenous activists, and corporations are actively inventing alternatives to consent out of the failed or unethical practices of the past.

POSTMEDICAL DEMANDS

One of the seemingly inherent ethical plateaus today is the problem of excess information and what to do with it. If one assumes that more information is inherently good or at least neutral, then the problem of too much information or a right *not* to know something seems paradoxical or nonsensical. Lindemann draws on classic sociological concepts, such as the Ego–Alter relationship, to look at how even death becomes a problematic demand because there are too many tests for it. Doctors, for instance, may struggle to tell a plausible, coherent, "gestalt" story of a situation that takes into account all the current information about it. But this gestalt is fragile to the extent that other tests (with their own risks of false positives and negatives) may suggest a different narrative. This is not simply a problem of getting better information, Lindemann suggests, but a product of the fact that "[i]n order to carry out a lab test, the gestalt has to be divided into parts which have to be compatible with the laboratory." This sociotechnical anatomy of discrete, incomplete, probabilistic parts is both more flexible and more refractory to coherence. In the United States, for instance, the proliferation of information opens doors to lawsuits in almost all poor medical outcomes, further driving the proliferation of as many tests as possible. As outlined earlier, a similar proliferation of evidence without coherence pervades Alzheimer's research. Even the strong correlations of plaques and tangles with dementia that promise correlation must take into account clear counter-examples, that is, people with clear plaques but no symptoms, and the converse.

Partial and contradictory evidence also pervades self-care, as Mol and Law discover when they follow postmedical demands in the everyday life of patients who must manage hypoglycemia. Their focus is not on noncompliant patients but on the very difficulty, if not impossibility, of proper maintenance. Measuring, feeling, injecting, waiting, shopping, running, and eating are all doing bodies. Despite ideal goals provided by medicine, bodies can be in tension with both life and themselves, one part of the body against another. People who "know" what to do, who act *after* medicine, are therefore constantly uncertain.

Another part of Lock's broad ethnographic project concerns the interaction of the intense demand for evidence with which to do something with the crisis in gathering good evidence given the moving target of the category itself. Looking at the long history of medicine, Tanner shows an always-present excessive demand for diagnosis and treatment. No part of medicine is immune from these postmedical demands—as in demands despite the fact that medicine can do no more. The current state of evidence is not enough for patients who want to be better. Understanding this allows us to follow Tanner in the consequences for studying biomedicine *as* culture and not commit two very easy and ready fallacies: first, the reduction of improper medicine to improper culture and, second, blaming contemporary biomedicine's excess solely on either corporate profit or state governmentality. In a different vein, Rose points out how medicine is reframed as a search for biovalue and the consequent relations between science and private corporations are powerful contexts for most contemporary biomedical practices. What all of these authors are pointing to is the inherent variability of life, health, and medicine. Very schematically, we can trace this variability as follows:

1. There are no simple means of evaluating possible medical solutions. They require balancing population definitions, effects, side effects, time, cost, impositions, obligations, and long-term effects. The weighting and interpretation of these are not determinate from research and clinical trial results alone. Just as individuals faced with a gamble will decide differently, so too will decision-making bodies.
2. The very definition of health is as difficult to decide as is that of normality. Even within any definable culture or society, there are various notions of health and normality that compete according to whether they should be optimal, ideal, sustainable, traditional, and profitable.
3. As many of the authors point out, so-called evidence-based medicine, whose promise is to resolve these issues, in fact adds to them because it faces the same inherent problems of deciding how to decide on the "proper" criteria for evaluation. Problems of participatory design are present in each step of an evaluation process.

POSTINDIVIDUAL BIOKNOWLEDGE

What many of these essays offer are accounts and insights into experimental solutions to this excess of demand and partial evidence: experimental at the level of management of relations to data, and experimental in terms of reception. Beck illustrates this precisely with the staging of a meeting between marrow donors and recipients in Cyprus in which the groups know that they have exchanged marrow, but no one knows just whose marrow went into whose body. Beck explains how this form of collective giving and reception is a management technique to moderate responsibility and prevent too much kinship from developing between individuals, and to prevent too much weight hanging on individual successes and failures. This management is opposite from in the United States, where individual bonds are celebrated. Each form of relation has its entailments. In the Cypriot case, we see an interesting production of a social relation, what Beck calls an "epistemic space of histocompatibility," in which a form of generalized exchange takes place that is not commodity exchange. The exchangers, too, enter into a novel kind of kinship, connected by what we might call a partial responsibility.

The struggle to incorporate genetic results, partial probabilities, and preventative strategies into one's life involves an experimental search for metaphors on the side of subjects as well as by doctors and researchers. Lock, and Duden and Samerski, engage in thick ethnographic discussions with risk-diagnosed patients. Perhaps not surprisingly, gene information is not so persuasive, especially if it contradicts one's life experiences with particular diseases or deaths. As Lock puts it, genetic risk estimates were fit into existing Alzheimer's disease experiences. Of course, genes are potent objects to think with. Whatever one's views, the ideas of hereditary transmission and genetic results are powerful, but *how* one lives with this information is not simply manageable.

However, as Lemke and Taussig are careful to note, it is not always up to the individual to interpret or incorporate risk information. Lemke examines a series of U.S. court decisions to show how troubling genetic risk can be, precisely because individual autonomy is supposed to be preserved. At issue is whether genetic information becomes obligatory because it is needed in order to be an autonomous individual. On these grounds, if information on one's genetic risk exists, it seems to be criminal for anyone not to tell the individual. This could be said to be equal to withholding information vital to one's health and life. Similarly, once informed, one can then be construed as having the obligation to inform all of one's kin (as in genetic relations) of their relative risk. Lemke's suggestion is that this form of interpretation is increasingly not about subjective decisions. You have no right not to know, but an extended obligation to first know your own risks, and second to do something about them.

Taussig traces a similar erosion of the individual in the presumption of consent in complete research trials where there is biological material preserved and where subjects, even dead ones, are assumed to have auto-consented to new forms of research on their DNA on the grounds that they would have if DNA research had existed then and if they had been asked. The issue today is the ethical plateau of the indetermination of this information. The logics of obligation are based on the idealized assumption that genes map clearly onto probabilities and meanings, and that bodies can be configured to match those meanings even if neither patients nor researchers buy this assumption.

Rose's analysis of the extension of the remit of biomedicine—beyond the boundaries set by diseases and their treatments to the management of susceptibilities and life itself—similarly turns on the transformation of responsibilities in the wake of emergent forms of bio-knowledge. The contradiction between the apparent individualization of "personalized medicine" and its products for profit challenges existing forms of both self-knowledge and obligation. But as this book as a whole demonstrates, the developments analyzed by Rose are taking place within "biomedicine as culture." Postgenomic, postmedical, postindividual plateaus are being lived today within biomedicine precisely as experimental forms of life.

REFERENCES

Beaulieu, Anne. 2001. Voxels in the brain: Neuroscience, informatics and changing notions of objectivity. *Social Studies of Science* 31, no. 5: 635–80.

Fischer, Michael M. J. 2003. *Emergent forms of life and the anthropological voice.* Durham, NC: Duke University Press.

Fox Keller, Evelyn. 2000. *The century of the gene.* Cambridge, MA: Harvard University Press.

Rheinberger, Hans-Jörg. 1997. *Toward a history of epistemic things: Synthesizing proteins in the test tube.* Stanford, CA: Stanford University Press.

Roberts, Elizabeth. 1998. "Native" narratives of connectedness: Surrogate motherhood and technology. In *Cyborg babies: From techno-sex to techno-tots,* edited by Robbie Davis-Floyd and Joseph Dumit, 193–211. London: Routledge.

Contributors

Stefan Beck is an assistant professor of European ethnology at the Humboldt-University, Berlin, and was a visiting assistant professor at the University of California, Berkeley, in 2000. He is currently working on different research projects focusing on social anthropology, the life sciences, and management and public health. He is the author of *Umgang mit Technik. Kulturelle Praxen und kulturwissenschaftliche Forschungskonzepte* (Akademie-Verlag, 1997); and the coeditor of *Körperpolitik—Biopolitik* (with Michi Knecht; Sonderheft Berliner Blätter, 2003), and *Surviving Globalization? Perspectives for the German Economic Model* (with Frank Klobes and Christoph Scherrer; Springer, 2005).

Regula Valérie Burri is an associated research fellow at Collegium Helveticum, Swiss Federal Institute of Technology (ETH) and University of Zurich. Her doctoral thesis, "Doing Images: Zur Praxis medizinischer Bilder" (forthcoming), explores the social and cultural implications of medical imaging. She has been a Swiss National Science Foundation research fellow and holds appointments with several Swiss universities. Her research interests focus on the relationship between science, technology, and society. She is the coauthor of "Social Studies of Scientific Images and Visualization," in Ed Hackett et al., *The Handbook of Science and Technology Studies* (with Joseph Dumit; MIT Press, 2007).

Barbara Duden is a trained social historian and teaches in the Sociology Department of Hannover University. She is the author of a large number of publications that examine "the body" as a historical category, in particular of *The Woman beneath the Skin* (Harvard University Press, 1991); *Disembodying Women: Perspectives on Pregnancy and the Unborn* (Harvard University Press, 1993); *Die Gene im Kopf—der Fötus im Bauch: Historisches zum Frauenkörper* (Hannover Offizin, 2002); and *Anatomie der Guten Hoffnung: Bilder vom ungeborenen Menschen 1500–1800* (Campus, 2005). Her current project, on which she is collaborating with Silja Samerski, explores the social and cultural effects of the "release of genetic terms" into everyday language.

Joseph Dumit is an associate professor in the Department of Anthropology and the director of the program in Science and Technology Studies at University of California, Davis. His research interests are the anthropology of science, technology, and medicine; medical anthropology; and social studies. He is the author of *Picturing Personhood: Brain Scans and Biomedical Identity* (Princeton University Press, 2004); and the coeditor of *Cyborgs & Citadels: Anthropological Interventions in Emerging Sciences and Technologies* (with Gary L. Downey; SAR Press, 1997), and *Cyborg Babies: From Techno-Sex to Techno-Tots* (with Robbie Davis-Floyd; Routledge, 1998). Dumit is the associate editor of the journal *Culture, Medicine & Psychiatry*.

John Law is a professor and acting cohead of the Department of Sociology at Lancaster University, and a former director of Lancaster University's Centre for Science Studies. His publications include *After Method: Mess in Social Science Research* (Routledge, 2004); *Aircraft Stories: Decentering the Object in Technoscience* (Duke University Press, 2002); *Complexities: Social Studies of Knowledge Practices* (coedited with Annemarie Mol; Duke University Press, 2002); *Actor Network Theory and After* (coedited with John Hassard; Blackwell Publishers, 1999); and *Organizing Modernity* (Blackwell Publishers, 1994). He was a coeditor of a special issue of *Society and Space*, "Boundaries: Materialities, Difference and Continuities" (with Annemarie Mol; 2005).

Thomas Lemke is a senior fellow in sociology at the University of Wuppertal and a fellow of the Institut für Sozialforschung, Frankfurt am Main. His current research project focuses on the concept of genetic risk and the social consequences of genetic diagnosis. He is the author of *Eine Kritik der politischen Vernunft—Foucaults Analyse der modernen Gouvernementalität* (Hamburg, Berlin Argument, 1997), *Veranlagung und Verantwortung. Genetische Diagnostik zwischen Selbstbestimmung und Schicksal* (Bielefeld transcript, 2004), and *Polizei der Gene. Formen und Felder genetischer Diskriminierung* (Campus, 2006); and the editor of *Michel Foucault: Analytik der Macht* (Suhrkamp, 2005).

Gesa Lindemann is an affiliated research fellow in the Department of Sociology at the Technical University Berlin. She received her PhD from the University of Bremen with a thesis on gender constructions. She was a visiting professor at the Universities of Munich and Bielefeld. Her recent books include *Die Grenzen des Sozialen. Zur sozio-technischen Konstruktion von Leben und Tod in der Intensivmedizin* (München Fink Verlag, 2002); and *Beunruhigende Sicherheiten. Zur Genese des Hirntodkonzepts* (Konstanz Universitätsverlag, 2003). Her current research is a comparative project on neuroscientific concepts of consciousness in human and animal research.

Margaret Lock is the Marjorie Bronfman Professor in Social Studies in Medicine, and is affiliated with the Department of Social Studies of Medicine and the Department of Anthropology at McGill University. She is a fellow of the Royal Society of Canada and an Officier de L'Ordre national du Québec. Her monographs include *East Asian Medicine in Urban Japan* (University of California Press, 1980*); Encounters with Aging: Mythologies of Menopause in Japan and North America* (University of California Press, 1993); and *Twice Dead: Organ Transplants and the Reinvention of Death* (University of California Press, 2002). Her books have received numerous prizes. She has edited or coedited ten other books and written over 160 scholarly articles. Her current research is concerned with postgenomic biology and its impact in the clinic, among families, and in society at large.

Annemarie Mol is Socrates Professor of Political Philosophy at the University of Twente, the Netherlands. She is the author of *The Body Multiple: Ontology in Medical Practice* (Duke University Press, 2002), which received the Ludwik Fleck Prize of the Society for the Social Studies of Science in 2004. Mol is the editor of *Complexities: Social Studies of Knowledge Practices* (with John Law; Duke University Press, 2002); *Differences in Medicine: Unraveling Practices, Techniques, and Bodies* (with Marc Berg; Duke University Press, 1998); and a special issue of *Society and Space*, "Boundaries: Materialities, Difference and Continuities" (with John Law; 2005). She is the author of "Proving or Improving: On Health Care Research as a Form of Self-Reflection," *Qualitative Health Research* 16, no. 3: 405–14.

Nelly Oudshoorn is professor in Technology Dynamics and Health Care at the University of Twente, the Netherlands. She is the author of *Beyond the Natural Body: An Archeology of Sex Hormones* (Routledge, 1994); and *The Male Pill: A Biography of a Technology in the Making* (Duke University Press, 2003). Together with Ann Saetnan and Marta Kirejczyk, she edited *Bodies of Technology: Women's Involvement with Reproductive Technologies* (Ohio University Press, 2000); and, together with Trevor Pinch, *How Users Matter: The Co-construction of Users and Technology* (MIT Press, 2003). Her current research focuses on the construction of trust in the design and use of telemonitoring technologies for cardiac patients.

Nikolas Rose is professor of sociology, convenor of the Department of Sociology, and director of the BIOS Centre for the Study of Bioscience, Biomedicine, Biotechnology and Society at the London School of Economics and Political Science. His books include *The Psychological Complex* (Routledge, 1984); *Inventing Ourselves* (Cambridge University Press, 1996); *Governing the Soul* (2nd ed., Free Associations, 1989); *Powers of Freedom: Reframing Political Thought* (Cambridge University Press, 1999) and *The Politics of Life Itself* (Princeton University Press, 2006). He is managing editor of *Economy and Society* and joint editor of *BioSocieties: An Interdisciplinary Journal for Social Studies of Neuroscience, Genomics, and the Life Sciences*. His current research concerns biological and genetic psychiatry and behavioral neuroscience, and its social, ethical, cultural, and legal implications.

Silja Samerski is a geneticist and social scientist in the Department of Sociology and Social Psychology at the University of Hannover. Together with Barbara Duden, she has been working on a project that investigated the ways "genes" and genetics are talked about in everyday conversations. Taking the example of genetic counseling, Samerski is interested in the implications that expert advice has for individuals and investigates how these individuals are transformed into managerial decision makers on their own behalf. Samerski is the author of *Die verrechnete Hoffnung: Von der selbstbestimmten Entscheidung durch genetische Beratung* (Münster, 2002).

Cornelius Schubert holds a PhD in sociology from the Technical University Berlin, where he works and teaches as a senior fellow in the Department of Sociology. He has effected ethnographic studies on time management practices in hospital wards and on the sociotechnical practices in operating rooms in Germany and Australia. His doctoral thesis, "Die Technik operiert mit. Sozio-technische Konstellationen bei der Arbeit" (Berlin, 2005), is concerned with distributed actions in hospital settings. His research interests are organizational studies, the ethnography of work, the sociology of medicine, and science and technology studies.

André Somers holds a Master degree in Philosophy of Science, Technology and Society from the University of Twente, the Netherlands. For his thesis, he studied the construction of user images by patient organizations as nontraditional designers of technology. He is currently working as a junior researcher at the Netherlands Centre for Science System Assessment at the Rathenau Institute in The Hague, the Netherlands. His current research focuses on the social aspects of the construction of large scale ICT-based knowledge and data sharing infrastructures and their effects on the communities they are imposed on.

Jakob Tanner is a professor for modern history at the Research Institute for Social and Economic History at the University of Zurich and a permanent fellow at the Collegium Helveticum, Swiss Federal Institute of Technology (ETH) and University of Zurich. He was a visiting professor at Bielefeld University and a fellow at the Institute for Advanced Study in Berlin, and was named a member of the Independent Commission of Experts Switzerland—Second World War by the Swiss government. His publications include *Fabrikmahlzeit* (Chronos, 1999); *Physiologie und industrielle Gesellschaft* (with Philipp Sarasin; Suhrkamp, 1998); *Historische Anthropologie* (Junius Verlag, 2004); and *Attraktion und Abwehr: Die Amerikanisierung der Alltagskultur in Europa* (with Angelika Linke; Böhlau, 2006).

Karen-Sue Taussig holds a joint appointment of assistant professor in the Departments of Anthropology and Medicine at the University of Minnesota. Her current project examines the diverse contexts in which people are learning new genetic knowledge and the way in which they incorporate and make sense of this knowledge in their everyday lives. She is the coauthor of "Flexible Eugenics: Technologies of the Self in the Age of Genetics," in A. Goodman, S. Lindee, and D. Heath's *Genetic Nature/Culture: Anthropology in the Age of Genetics, Genetics in the Age of Anthropology* (University of California Press, 2003); and "Genealogical Dis-Ease: Where Hereditary Abnormality, Biomedical Explanation and Family Responsibility Meet," in S. McKinnon and S. Franklin's *Relative Values: Reconfiguring Kinship Studies* (with Rayna Rapp and Deborah Heath; Duke University Press, 2001).

Index

Printed in the United States
by Baker & Taylor Publisher Services